Techniques of measurement in medicine: 2
Series Editor: Professor B. Watson
Department of Medical Electronics
St Bartholomew's Hospital, London
Consultant Editor: Professor J. Rotblat

Electromedical instrumentation — a guide
for medical personnel

W0114547

Electromedical instrumentation

A GUIDE FOR MEDICAL PERSONNEL

P. BERGVELD

Department of Electrical Engineering
Twente University of Technology
Enschede, The Netherlands

Cambridge University Press

CAMBRIDGE

LONDON   NEW YORK   NEW ROCHELLE

MELBOURNE   SYDNEY

CAMBRIDGE UNIVERSITY PRESS
Cambridge, New York, Melbourne, Madrid, Cape Town,
Singapore, São Paulo, Delhi, Tokyo, Mexico City

Cambridge University Press
The Edinburgh Building, Cambridge CB2 8RU, UK

Published in the United States of America by Cambridge University Press, New York

www.cambridge.org
Information on this title: www.cambridge.org/9780521293051

First published 1980
Re-issued 2011

A catalogue record for this publication is available from the British Library

Library of Congress Cataloguing in Publication data

Bergveld, P. 1940–
Electromedical instrumentation

(Techniques of measurement in medicine; 2)
Includes index
1. Medical electronics. 1. Title. 11. Series.
(DNLM: 1. Electronics, Medical–Instrumentation.
2. Biomedical engineering – Instrumentation.
QT34 B499e)
R856.B43   610'.28   77-85711

ISBN 978-0-521-21892-4 Hardback
ISBN 978-0-521-29305-1 Paperback

Contents

Foreword

A simple introduction to electronic engineering had to be included in this series because many new clinical measurement techniques involve the use of electronic equipment. However, if electronic techniques are described without close reference to the medical instrumentation, it can be difficult for nurses and doctors to become interested enough to read and absorb a subject which is foreign to their previous experience. This book evolved from a course of lectures which Dr Bergveld gave to nurses, and should be easy reading for medical personnel with little knowledge of physics or mathematics.

The relevance of each topic should be easily appreciated because the examples used to illustrate the engineering principles are taken from medical electronics instruments used for measurement in clinical situations.

It is my hope that this book will be of use in training doctors, nurses and technicians to appreciate the mode of operation of electronic equipment found today in a modern hospital and enable them to use it more effectively without stress to themselves or to the patients.

B.W. Watson

Preface

Owing to the increasing use of electronic instrumentation in medical practice, it is desirable that medical and nursing personnel have some technical knowledge of electronic equipment. In the first place they must be able to decide whether a piece of electronic equipment should or should not be used. Advantages have to be balanced against disadvantages, and the best equipment chosen in each case. Secondly, the user of the equipment must have mastered the necessary operating skill in order to realise its full potential. Last but not least, especially when using electrical apparatus, the patient's safety must be guaranteed.

It is the aim of this book to help those members of the medical profession who meet these three problems but did not come in contact with electronic instrumentation during their training.

The author is aware of the breadth of the area covered by available instrumentation and the large numbers of types of each specific instrument. It is impossible to review all these types of instrument. However, there are only a limited number of basic principles and methods used in electromedical instruments, and experience in teaching doctors and nurses has shown that a knowledge of principles, allied to a careful reading of manufacturers' instructions, enables users to understand the operation of most instruments. In this book the reader will find a survey of basic principles and methods, with illustrations of the applications in the most common fields of medical practice, for instance the registration of cardiac activity by means of the ECG. More complicated instrumental systems, such as those used for intensive care, are discussed in the light of the basic principles. These include acquaintance with three important concepts in electricity: voltage, current and resistance.

A basic knowledge of some electrical phenomena is essential, and this book will begin with chapters concerning them. Explanations and illustrations have been chosen to be as close as possible to the daily practice of the reader. This basic knowledge is necessary for the understanding of the last, probably the most important, chapter of this book, concerning the safety of patients connected to electromedical instrumentation.

This book has been written for both individual study and for use in courses in which the various methods of application are described on the basis of a given principle and can be demonstrated with apparatus.

The author hopes that this book will be helpful to all those who use electrical equipment to treat ill people and often save their lives.

Enschede, The Netherlands   Dr Piet Bergveld

1. Introduction

As a starting point, it is important to ask whether the use of technical equipment, or more specifically the application of electro-medical instrumentation in medical practice, will have a significant bearing on patient care; and if so, in which cases can this be to the greatest advantage. The development of electronic apparatus in medical practice is more than a mere manifestation of the trend towards the increasing use of electrical equipment in modern life. The application of electronic equipment in medical practice can raise standards of medical care. This can best be illustrated by considering the following points.

Electronic instrumentation can be used in the objective recording of symptoms where observation, using the senses, may provide much information about a patient's condition; often, unfortunately, such methods of collecting data are far from accurate. For these reasons, additional methods of observation have been developed, offering great advantages in accuracy, discrimination and response time.

It will be obvious that the availability of reliable technical equipment, in this case for physiological measurement, is of considerable importance and may be preferred to human abilities when reliability and accuracy are of paramount importance. An example of this is in monitoring of a patient.

During the recording of symptoms, it is necessary to carry out comparisons with previous data, and also to discuss the symptoms with other people. For skilful and accurate recording, electrical equipment can offer great advantages. Examples of this are in the recording of the ECG, and the motion of the mitral valve cusps using ultrasound.

The interpretation of observed and recorded symptoms can be done visually, but again by the use of electronic equipment this may be done much more accurately and in much more detail. A variety of systems, from rather simple single-purpose instruments up to the most complicated computer systems, may be used. The result of signal processing, as it is called, may help medical staff to diagnose conditions more precisely, resulting in decisions to take more appropriate measures. An extreme example is the decision to use an electronic defibrillator immediately after ventricular fibrillation is recognised. In this case the ease with which the condition may be detected using electronic equipment is clearly of great advantage.

The modification of the function of certain organs may be necessary if it appears that the normal limits have been exceeded.

This may indicate medical or surgical treatment, or the use of electrical equipment, such as the implantation of a pacemaker.

The processes of measuring, recording, interpretation and functional adjustment are often carried out in medical practice as a closed circuit, although the various stages of the process may not always be recognised separately. A conversation between a doctor and a patient, and the corresponding investigation in the clinical laboratory (observation and interpretation), followed by a recommended diet (adjustment) is a simple example of such a process. An example in which most stages of this process are carried out by electronic instruments may be found in an intensive care unit. In order to get an insight into such a closed circuit process, it is useful to make a schematic representation called a block diagram (as is often done in technology).

It is the aim of this book to deal with the principles and applications of the electronic devices which are commonly used to carry out the specific functions of the various blocks of Fig. 1.1.

In the processes of measuring, recording, interpretation and adjustment the reliability of the different functional units is of great importance. The final diagnosis must always be made by skilled medical staff, and they have to be absolutely sure that they can rely on the operation of the instruments used. The readings of the instruments have to provide the user with relevant information of medical significance without artifacts. A measurement of, for instance, the electrical activity of the heart may be disturbed by other electrical sources within or outside the body.

It is not necessary to provide the medical user with data displayed with more accuracy than the normal spread of biological

Fig. 1.1. A schematic representation or block diagram of the closed-circuit process of patient care.

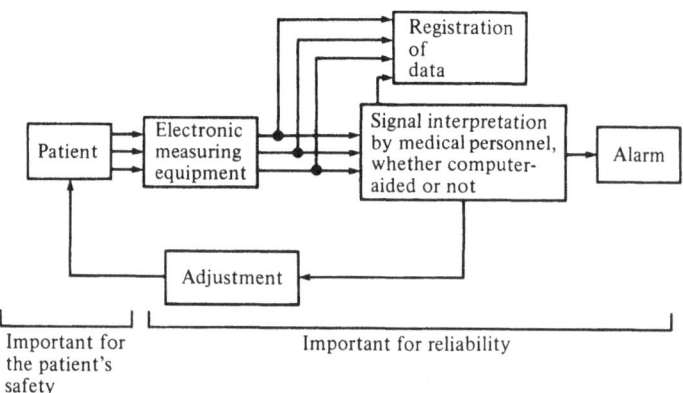

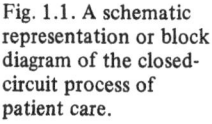
Important for the patient's safety

Important for reliability

parameters. A measured heart rate with a mean value of 120 beats per minute is accurate enough; information giving 120.5 or even 120 ± 1 is, in this case, of no advantage in making a diagnosis. A temperature measurement of ± 0.1 °C is good enough for most purposes.

Besides the requirements of reliability and accuracy of the equipment, the safety requirements are even more important. In addition to the safe construction of the equipment, a requirement expected to be fulfilled by the manufacturer, the equipment must also be used in such a way that accidents cannot occur. This is the responsibility of the user. The last chapter is a helpful guide for a safe application of electromedical instrumentation. First, however, some basic electrical concepts must be understood, and this information is provided in the first few chapters. Safety rules are also mentioned at relevant points in the text, because the significance of this subject as an important aspect of routine work cannot be over-emphasised.

2. The electric potential

Everyone knows that an object will fall towards the ground if it is dropped. In general, it can be asserted that free objects always fall from a higher level to a lower one. In this case, movement from high to low is due to the force of gravity, but there are also other forces known in nature which cause movement from higher to lower levels. One of these is the electrical force, which propels electrical charges from higher to lower levels, called, in this case, higher and lower *electrical potentials.*

Some electrical phenomena were known to the early Egyptians, who discovered electricity in their experiences with electric fish. The ancient Greeks found that certain electrical phenomena could be generated by rubbing amber with a woollen cloth. Light objects, such as small pieces of paper, were attracted by the rubbed amber. Today it is known that other materials too show this amber-like behaviour and can attract light objects after being rubbed. The same effect occurs when combing dry hair. This effect is now called 'electrostatic attraction', after *electron*, the Greek word for amber.

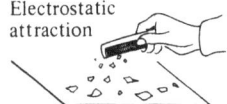

Fig. 2.1. An experiment illustrating electrostatic attraction.

It is now also known that as a result of rubbing certain materials, such as nylon, electrical charges are created which will attract each other after they are mechanically separated. The electrical potential of one of the rubbed materials is higher than that of the other.

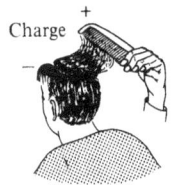

Fig. 2.2. Electrostatic attraction, accompanied by discharging and crackling sounds of tiny sparks.

The material with a higher potential has a surplus of positive electrical charges, while the material with the lower electrical potential has a deficit of positive electrical charges. Hence positive charges will tend to flow from a higher electrical potential to a lower electrical potential. A deficit of positive charges can also be seen as a surplus of negative charges. One can therefore assert that positive charges will move from a positive electrical potential to a negative electrical potential, indicating that a positive potential is higher than a negative potential. The tendency for positive charges to move from an object with a positive electrical potential to an object with a negative electrical potential will be the greater the more positive the positive potential is, and the more negative the negative potential is. In other words, if the potential difference between two objects is increased, the electrical force on the charges also increases. This force can be so high that the charges will jump through the air from the object with the higher potential to the object with the lower potential; this is called discharge. During a thunderstorm very high electrical potentials are built up inside clouds — a flash of lightning is nothing more than a large electrical discharge. Fortunately, such high electrical potentials are not encountered in electrical equipment in everyday use, but we must still be aware of their effects.

As already mentioned, nylon clothing can also be easily charged by rubbing against other materials. The subsequent attraction to other fabrics can be troublesome, and it may be dangerous if, as is often the case, discharge through the air also occurs. Often, someone wearing nylon clothing can hear the crackle of tiny sparks and, in a dark room, can see these sparks. These sparks are caused by static electricity, and may occur with certain floor coverings as well as clothing; sparks can be extremely dangerous if they occur in operating theatres where inflammable liquids and gases are used. It seems that static electricity cannot be adequately controlled, so the only safe procedure is to forbid the use of materials which have static-electrical behaviour in operating theatres and places of potential danger.

Coming back to electricity itself, the points made earlier may be summarised by the statement that objects may have a positive potential or a negative potential and that positive charges tend to move 'downhill' towards a lower potential. In other words, positive charges are repelled by objects with a positive potential and attracted by those with a negative potential. The same rule applies to negative charges; negative charges are repelled by a negative potential and attracted by a positive one. The smallest amount of negative charge which can move from a negative to a positive potential is that carried by an electron. The significance of electron transport will be explained in detail in Chapter 3. First the concept of electrical potential will be dealt with more fully.

As already mentioned, the electrical potential of an object is always defined with respect to the potential of another object, either more positive or more negative, or with respect to an object which has no electrical potential (Fig. 2.3). Electrical potential is measured in volts, abbreviated as V, and the electrical

Fig. 2.3. A schematic representation of the concepts of potential and voltage.

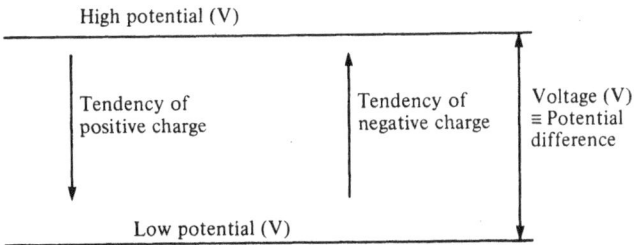

High potential (V)

Tendency of positive charge

Tendency of negative charge

Voltage (V) ≡ Potential difference

Low potential (V)

potential of the earth is conventionally assumed to be zero. An object may thus have a potential with respect to earth of, for instance, + 10 V, + 100 V, − 0.1 V etc. In practice the potential difference between two objects, or an object and earth, is the important quantity. This is called voltage (also expressed in volts). In Fig. 2.4, for example, object A has a potential of + 10 V with respect to earth, object B, + 100 V, and object C, − 1 V; the voltage (A−earth) is + 10 V; (B−earth) is + 100 V; (C−earth) is − 1 V; (earth−B) is − 100 V; (A−B) is − 90 V; (A−C) is + 11 V etc.

As already mentioned, one method of generating a voltage between two materials is to rub them together. The electricity made in this way is not usable, however, because after the discharge the voltage will drop to zero. Scientists therefore looked for means to generate voltages which would be available for use over longer periods of time. One method was found around 1800 by Alexander Volta, from whose name the name 'volt' is derived. He found that a voltage is generated between two plates of different metals immersed in acid. The voltage is generated by electrochemical processes occurring between the metal plate and the acid. Such materials are called galvanic elements, after Luigi Galvani who first experimented with them around 1770, without, however, suspecting their possible applications. This principle is now widely used, for instance in car batteries, called accumulators. Here, two metal plates are immersed in an acid, usually sulphuric acid. One of the plates, which are called poles, is positive with respect to the other. This is indicated on the battery as + pole (called the anode), and −− pole (called the cathode).

Recently, miniature accumulators have been developed; these are sealed in such a way that the acid cannot evaporate. Such accumulators do not need to be refilled with distilled water, as

Fig. 2.4. Examples of various voltages.

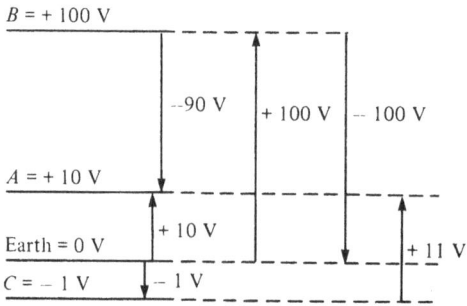

unsealed types do, and are often used in battery-operated medical
equipment. Instruments powered by a battery are useful when
safety requirements are very high; the reason for this will be
explained further in Chapter 12.

The electrochemical processes which occur at a metal–liquid
interface may cease as one of the ingredients becomes exhausted,
so that after a period of time the voltage between the poles drops.
Fortunately, the electrochemical processes can be reversed by
applying a current to the accumulator. By doing this, the accumulator can be recharged so that the original voltage between the
poles is again present and the accumulator can be re-used.

Another source of electrical potential is the dry battery or dry
cell, commonly used in transistor radios and torches (flashlights).
Here two poles can again be seen in the construction. One of the
poles, usually the negative one, forms the case of the cell, and the

Fig. 2.5. A schematic
representation of an
accumulator.

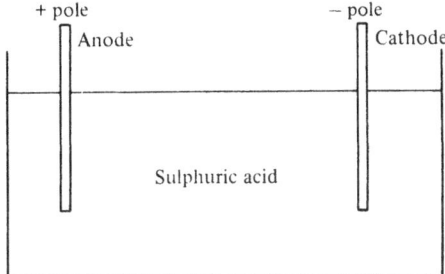

Fig. 2.6. Examples of a
12 V and a 6 V
accumulator, and the
symbol for an
accumulator.

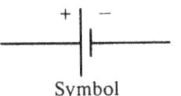

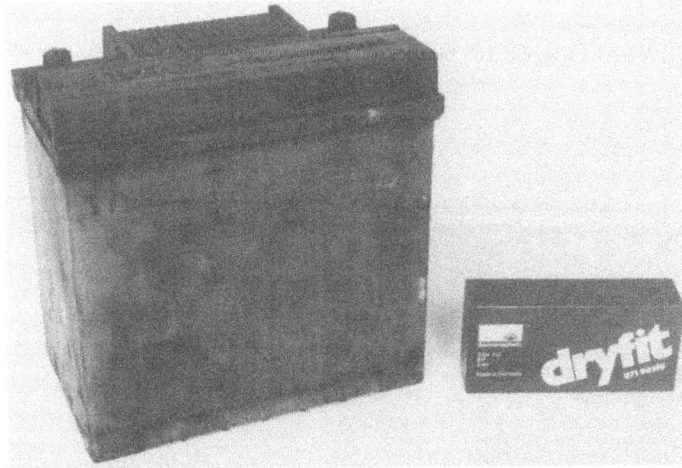

liquid between the metals is in the form of a jelly-like substance. In the dry battery, electrochemical processes again take place at the metals, which are 'consumed' as a direct result of these processes. This means that after a certain period of time, when the material of one pole has been exhausted, the voltage between the poles of the battery falls. The battery must then be thrown away; it cannot be recharged as the materials have been used up.

The maximum voltage which can be reached between the poles of an accumulator is approximately 2 V, and for a dry cell the maximum is 1.5 V. For higher voltages, more cells have to be

Fig. 2.7. Examples of various types of dry batteries.

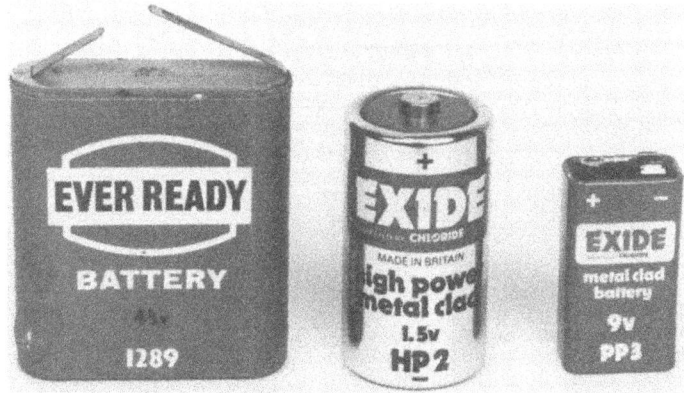

Fig. 2.8. A symbolic representation of three 1.5 V batteries or accumulators connected in series.

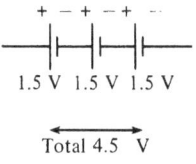

1.5 V 1.5 V 1.5 V

Total 4.5 V

Fig. 2.9. An open view of batteries in which it can be seen how, in reality, cells are connected in series: at the left-hand side by internal wires and at the right-hand side simply by piling the separate cells.

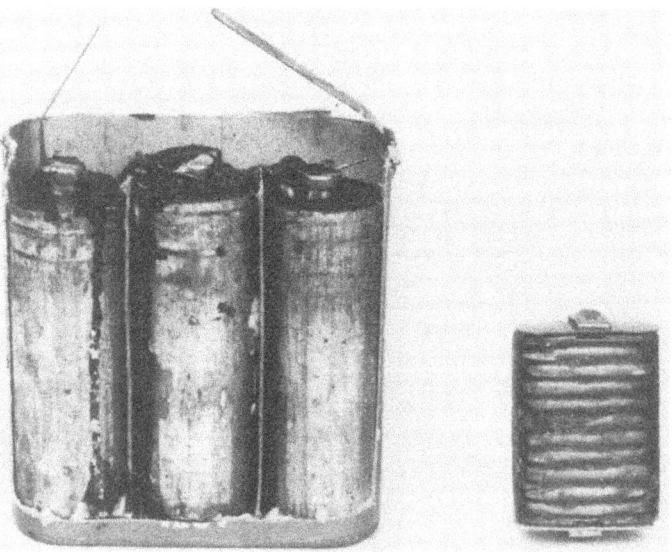

connected together in such a way that the total voltage of the connected cells is the sum of the separate cell voltages. This is called a series connection. The anode of one cell is connected to the cathode of a second cell and so on. A motor-cycle battery of 6 V consists of three cells of 2 V each, connected in series. This can sometimes be seen where the interconnections are made externally, and three filling caps may be distinguished. Similarly, a 12 V car battery consists of six cells connected in series and has six filling caps. A dry battery of 4.5 V consists of three dry cells of 1.5 V each. Removing the paper packing of such a battery will reveal the separate elements with the necessary interconnections.

A 9 V transistor radio battery consists of six elements each of 1.5 V, which are placed on top of each other, as can again be seen by removing the battery case.

Batteries can also be connected in such a way that together they generate a voltage which is equal to the voltage of each of the separate batteries. The positive poles are connected together, as are the negative poles. The result is that the compound battery can provide a voltage for a longer period of time because the surface area of the plates is now larger and it takes more time for electrochemical processes to exhaust the plates.

This type of interconnection of voltage sources (anode to anode and cathode to cathode) is called a parallel connection. In practice this option for increasing the lifetime of a battery is not often used; instead the same effect is achieved by batteries with larger plates.

Note that the basic principle of an accumulator or a battery is the generation of a voltage between a metal and an electrolyte. Similarly, a metal used as an electrode, such as an ECG electrode, will generate a voltage when it is in contact with a body fluid. This is termed the *electrode potential*. It can disturb the readings and measurements for which the electrodes are used. This problem is further dealt with in Chapter 6.

As already mentioned, it is always easy to distinguish the two poles of a battery, a positive pole and a negative pole, the polarity

Fig. 2.10. A symbolic representation of three 1.5 V batteries connected in parallel.

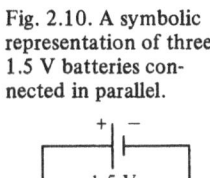
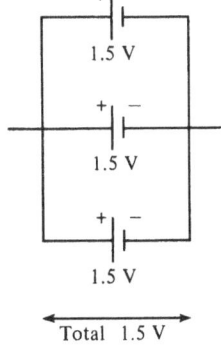

Fig. 2.11. A surface electrode in contact with body fluid behaves as a battery and thus creates a voltage, termed the electrode potential.

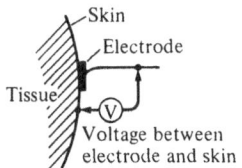

being determined by the plate materials used in the construction of the battery. This type of voltage is called a *direct voltage*, because the direction of the voltage between the two poles is always from + (highest potential) to − (lowest potential).

If the negative pole is connected to earth, which by definition has a potential of 0 V, then the free pole is positive with respect to earth. If the positive pole is connected to earth, then the free pole is negative with respect to earth. If one alternately opens and closes the connections to earth, then the free pole will alternately be positive and negative, which means, in the case of a 1.5 V battery, that the free pole would alternately be + 1.5 V and − 1.5 V. A voltage in which the polarity changes periodically is called an *alternating voltage*.

A disadvantage of batteries is that they cannot provide electrical voltages for long periods, as they soon become exhausted. Even if some varieties can be recharged, their limited period of use is a serious problem. As a result of this limitation, other processes have been investigated which would generate a voltage in an inexhaustible way. It was discovered that when a conducting wire, or a coil of conducting wire, was moved through the field around a magnet, an electric current flowed along the wire. This discovery is the basis of all dynamos and electricity generators. In practice the most convenient movement is rotational, and electricity is generated by the coil revolving through the magnetic field.

Fig. 2.12. A battery provides a direct voltage for a certain time.

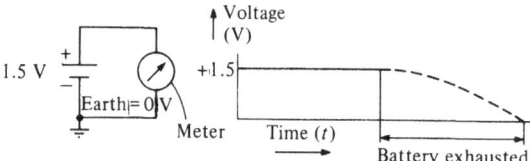

Fig. 2.13. The principle of creating an alternating voltage.

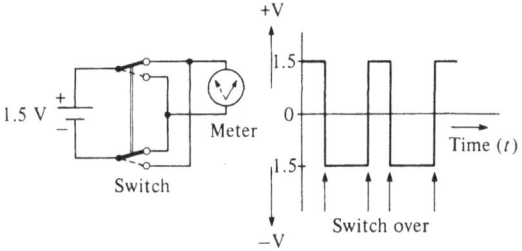

It should be noted that the electromagnetic effect mentioned above also works the other way around. A voltage connected to the ends of a coil causes the coil to move with respect to a magnetic field. In a rotating arrangement the coil or the magnet will then rotate. This is the principle of the electric motor.

Two poles can be distinguished in a dynamo, namely the two ends of the internal coil. When the coil rotates, after each half-turn the plane of the coil is opposite the plane of the magnet, while after a full turn they are again in the original position. The result is that the voltage generated between the ends of the coil changes its polarity every half-turn, thus providing an alternating voltage.

In electric power stations very large dynamos are used, producing alternating voltages up to 10 000 V. This voltage is transported by means of high-tension cables to transformer stations on the edges of cities and towns. Here the high voltage is transformed to a lower voltage (240 V, 220 V or 110 V). From these transformers it is again carried by means of wires or cables to power points in houses, factories and hospitals. This is why domestic power points provide an alternating voltage which can be used for most types of household electrical equipment. The voltage is available as long as the engines in the power stations are working.

Most electronic apparatus, however, requires a direct voltage for its operation. Thus, rectifiers have been developed which convert the alternating voltage of the mains to a direct voltage for use in electronic equipment. Instruments which can be used with a mains supply usually have a built-in transformer and rectifier. Some manufacturers deliver the transformer and rectifier parts of the equipment separately; this separate apparatus is called a power supply. Medical equipment is often manufactured with a separate

Fig. 2.14. A schematic representation of the principle of a dynamo, in which a coil rotates in a magnetic field.

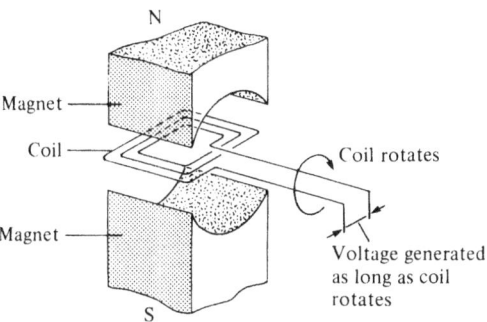

power supply; the advantage of this is that one power supply can be used for more than one instrument, thus reducing the total cost of the system.

Returning to the concept of alternating voltage, in which the polarity periodically fluctuates from positive to negative, it is important to know that various alternating waveforms can be distinguished. The most common waveforms are given descriptive names such as square-wave, triangular, sawtooth and sinusoidal.

Combinations of direct and alternating voltage are possible, for example a sinusoidal voltage may be combined with a direct voltage level. The polarity of such a voltage might then be always positive, but fluctuating periodically. A pulsating voltage pulse is an example of an alternating voltage, alternately positive and zero.

Human nerves and muscles generate voltages which can be measured using electrodes placed on the skin (see Chapter 8). These voltages are also alternating voltages with a recognisable waveform, for instance the electrocardiogram (ECG), electromyogram (EMG) and electroencephalogram (EEG). The ECG

Fig. 2.15. (a) A schematic representation of a power station, with high-tension cables, transformer and mains supply; (b) a sinusoidal alternating voltage of 240 V.

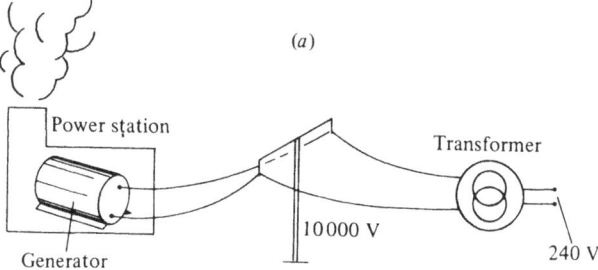

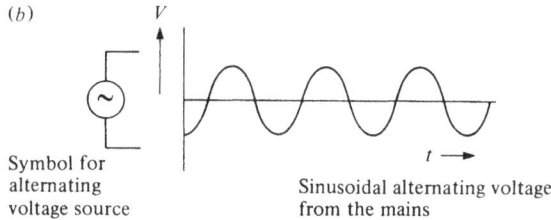

Fig. 2.16. A rectifier converts an alternating voltage into a direct voltage.

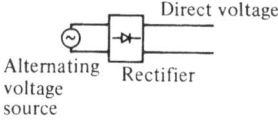

waveform is a manifestation of the electrical activity of the heart, the EMG of skeletal muscles, and the EEG of the brain. Deviations from the usual patterns may indicate abnormal activity at the

Fig. 2.17. Examples of alternating voltages.

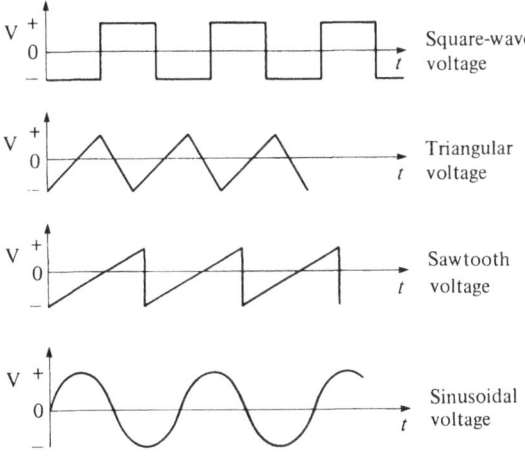

Square-wave voltage

Triangular voltage

Sawtooth voltage

Sinusoidal voltage

Fig. 2.18. Examples of alternating voltages superimposed on a direct voltage.

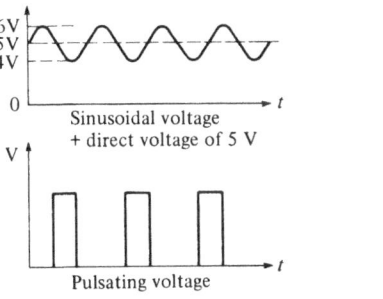

Sinusoidal voltage + direct voltage of 5 V

Pulsating voltage

Fig. 2.19. Examples of bio-electric voltages.

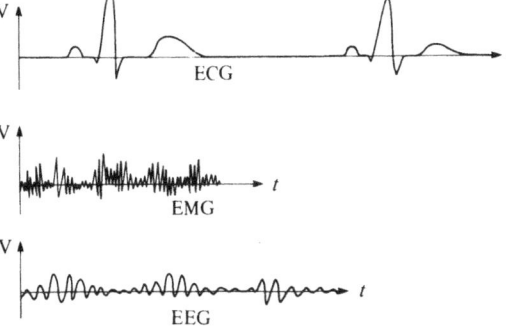

ECG

EMG

EEG

source of the signal – heart, muscle or brain, and indicate the need for treatment. Thus it is important to be able to record these biopotentials properly, as described in Chapter 8.

The waveforms of alternating voltages are always characterised by two main parameters, the *amplitude* and the *period*. The amplitude (A) of an alternating voltage is the maximum value with respect to 0 V (Fig. 2.20). The difference between the maximum positive and the maximum negative value is called the peak-to-peak value, which is thus $2A$ for a voltage symmetrical around 0 V (Fig. 2.20). The amplitude is expressed in volts (V), or in smaller parts: millivolts (mV), one thousandth of a volt; microvolts (μV), one millionth of a volt.

Most alternating voltages consist of one basic form, for instance one sine-wave, square, triangle, or ECG complex, which repeats itself as time proceeds. The repeat time is called the period, T, of the voltage waveform and is expressed in seconds (s), milliseconds (ms) or microseconds (μs).

The more frequently the characteristic waveform repeats itself within a certain time (i.e. the shorter the period, T) the greater is the repeating frequency, f. If, for instance, 50 periods occur every second (thus 1 period = 1/50 s = 0.02 s = 20 ms) then the frequency is 50 periods per second, also known as 50 cycles per second (50 c/s) or 50 hertz (50 Hz). This is in fact the frequency of the mains supply in Britain.

Increasing the frequency by a factor of 2 will decrease the period by a factor of 2. This relation can be written as follows: $f = 1/T$. For an ECG with, for instance, 60 beats per minute, which means that an ECG complex is generated every second, the characterising frequency is 1 Hz; with 120 beats per minute this frequency is 2 Hz.

To obtain an appreciation of the magnitude and frequency of some commonly used voltages, some of them are shown in Tables 2.1 and 2.2.

Table 2.1. *Magnitude of commonly occurring voltages*

Voltages used in		
nuclear physics	Megavolt (MV) = 1 000 000 V	= 10^6 volt
X-ray equipment	Kilovolt (kV) = 1000 V	= 10^3 volt
Batteries, accumulators	Volt (V) = 1 V	
ECG and EMG voltages	Millivolt (mV) = 0.001 V	= 10^{-3} volt
EEG voltages	Microvolt (μV) = 0.000001 V	= 10^{-6} volt

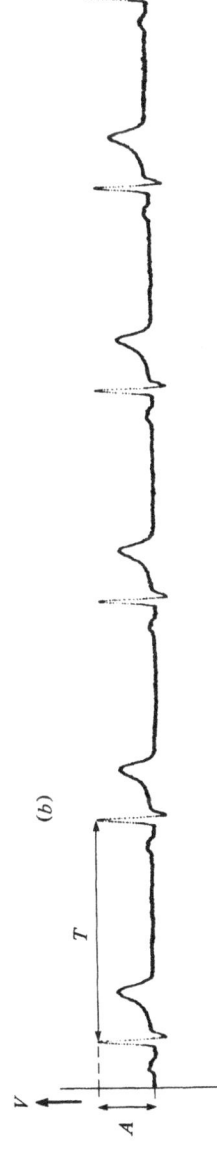

Fig. 2.20. (a) Any alternating voltage is characterised by its amplitude, A, and period, T. (b) Typical ECG registration, also characterised by the amplitude, A, and period, T.

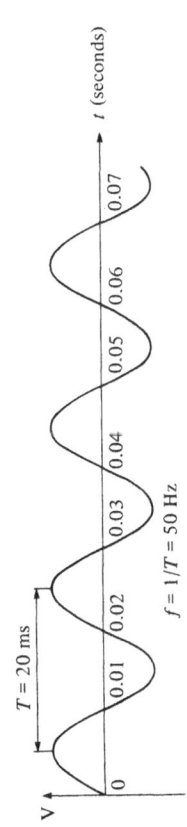

Fig. 2.21. The mains supply is an alternating voltage, with a frequency of 50 Hz in Britain.

As already mentioned, a voltage waveform may be the result of a combination of two or more voltages, for example a sinusoidal voltage on top of a direct voltage. In this case the amplitude of the resulting voltage is the sum of the amplitudes of the separate voltages added at each given moment. If two or more alternating voltages are added, the result is more difficult to describe, because these voltages can have a difference in their frequencies, as well as a difference in their amplitudes. The result is a waveform which usually differs greatly from the original waveforms, and is not simple to predict. In general, the frequency of the component with the lowest original frequency can be recognised easily, this is called the *base waveform*. Adding higher frequencies to a base waveform usually increases the slopes of the resulting waveform. The higher the frequencies added, the steeper the slopes of the waveform and the sharper the edges. In this way a square-shaped voltage with a repeating period of, say, 1 s (therefore with a basic frequency of 1 Hz) can originate from a sinusoidal voltage of 1 Hz to which a large number of voltages with higher frequencies have been added. The higher the frequencies of the added voltages, the sharper the square wave.

Although not a terminology used for characterising biomedical signals, technicians often express for practical purposes the voltage of an electrical signal as the effective value, the so-called root-mean-square value (abbreviated to r.m.s.). The r.m.s. value of a sinusoidal voltage with an amplitude of A is $A/\sqrt{2}$. The mains supply is always expressed as an r.m.s. value, i.e. 220/V r.m.s. This means that the actual amplitude of the mains supply is 220 $\times \sqrt{2} \approx 300$ V, periodically positive and negative, resulting in a peak-to-peak value of $2A \approx 600$ V!

Fig. 2.22. Base waveform with an added harmonic.

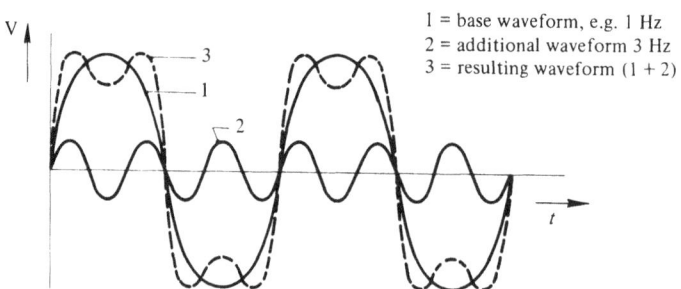

1 = base waveform, e.g. 1 Hz
2 = additional waveform 3 Hz
3 = resulting waveform (1 + 2)

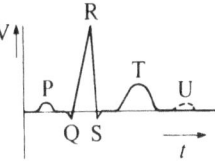

Fig. 2.23. Drawing of an ECG complex, consisting of a P, Q, R, S, T, and U-wave.

In general, each waveform, for instance an EEG signal or an ECG complex, can be divided into a base frequency and added higher frequencies. These more complex signals are characterised not by an amplitude and one frequency, but by an amplitude or peak-to-peak voltage and a frequency band or spectrum. This is shown in Table 2.2, where (for physiological signals) a frequency band is given.

Considering an ECG as an example, it is striking that the base frequency is of the order of 1 to 2 Hz and that each ECG complex consists of different pulse-shaped waveforms, due to many other frequency components. Consequently it appears that an ECG can be characterised by a certain frequency spectrum.

Cardiologists have given names to the various separate pulses, such as P-wave, QRS-complex and T-wave. They found that the P-wave originates from electrical activity of the atrium, the QRS from ventricle activity and the T-wave corresponds to the reverse process, the repolarisation of the cells.

Characteristic time intervals have been studied between the different waves with respect to each other and with respect to the previous or next corresponding similar wave. Also the shape of each separate wave is of interest and thus the frequency spectrum which determines the particular form. It appears that the ECG spectrum of frequencies lies within the 0.5 to 100 Hz band, and this means that the registration equipment, a recorder (see Chapter 9) or a monitor (see Chapter 10), must be able to measure all the frequencies produced. Should this not be the case, i.e. if certain frequency components are not recorded and are lost owing to inadequate equipment, the ECG waveform will be deformed, and an accurate diagnosis will not be possible. The more the

Table 2.2. *Frequencies of commonly occurring signals*

EEG voltages	0.5 Hz to 100 Hz
Repeating frequencies of ECG	0.3 Hz to 3 Hz
Tremor frequency	3 Hz to 10 Hz
Mains-supply frequency	50 or 60 Hz
Acoustical frequencies of the human voice	300 Hz to 3 kHz
Audible acoustical frequency	20 Hz to 15 kHz
Physiotherapeutic radiation equipment	1 MHz to 25 MHz
Frequency of visible light waves	0.38×10^{15} Hz to 0.79×10^{15} Hz

Fig. 2.24. (a) Drawing of an unfiltered ECG. (b) Drawing of a filtered ECG.

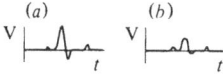

(a)   (b)

Fig. 2.25. Effect of filtering on a pulse-shaped voltage: (a) unfiltered; (b) less higher frequencies; (c) less lower frequencies.

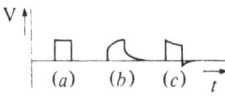

(a)   (b)   (c)

higher frequencies are filtered out of the spectrum (see Chapter 5) the more the sharper peaks are rounded off.

This effect is undesirable and therefore before each ECG recording is performed the equipment has to be assessed for its ability to record and register the necessary frequency-band. A very easy way to test this requirement is by using a calibration pulse. Such a test is often incorporated in the equipment in such a way that pushing a button connects a pulse-shaped voltage to the apparatus. This should be recorded as a very sharp pulse. If, however, owing to deterioration in the apparatus the higher frequencies are omitted, then the recorded pulse will show rounded edges. Alternatively, if the lower frequencies are not properly recorded, then the flat peak of the pulse will begin to sag. In both cases the recording apparatus has to be adjusted. More will be said about ECG recording in Chapter 8.

A similar description can be given of EEG recordings. EEG voltages also consist of internally added alternating voltages with different frequencies. The contributing frequencies are split up into certain frequency bands which are characteristic for normal brain activity and are called rhythms. The following rhythms can be distinguished:

α-rhythm (alpha) : 8–14 Hz
β-rhythm (beta) : 14–60 Hz
θ-rhythm (theta) : 4–8 Hz
δ-rhythm (delta) : <4 Hz

The amplitudes of these rhythms are inversely proportional to their frequency, and are of the order of a few microvolts. In an EEG recording the different rhythms appear mixed, so that the separate rhythms cannot be easily distinguished unless one of them is dominant. In general, however, the human eye cannot detect the contributing rhythms from a complex curve and therefore analysis requires additional observational tools, as already mentioned in Chapter 1. Frequency-spectrum analysers, which can analyse complex waveforms in terms of their component frequencies, are available. The use of a frequency-spectrum analyser in EEG analyses is a good example of how electronic apparatus can improve medical diagnosis by enhancing the human capability to discriminate between complicated signals.

In clinical practice there are often no 'clean voltages' available and signals such as EEG, ECG or EMG are available mixed with each other or other voltages generated in the same body. This problem will be further discussed in Chapter 5.

In some waveforms no special frequencies can be distinguished;
many frequencies contribute randomly. This type of voltage, generated by electrodes, electronic circuitry etc. is called noise. Most
recordings of physiological signals are slightly disturbed by the
noise of the electronic apparatus used to pick up these signals.

Potential differences occur on the surface and within the body,
and can be recorded for diagnostic purposes. These potential
differences, or biopotentials as they are called, may always be
characterised by their amplitude and frequency, or more usually
by a frequency spectrum. Many examples of these signals are given
in the following chapters.

Fig. 2.26. Typical EEG
waveforms.

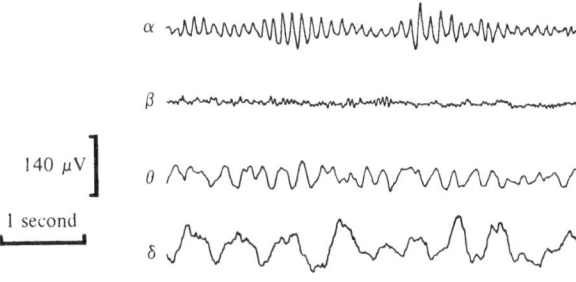

140 μV

1 second

Fig. 2.27. ECG regis-
trations disturbed by
EMG voltages.

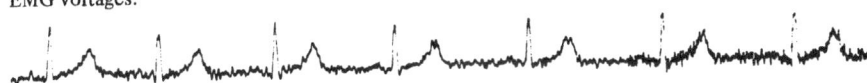

3. The electric current

As already mentioned in the previous chapter, the smallest amount of negative charge which can move from a negative to a positive potential is that carried by an electron. Electrons can only move if there is a fairly easy path to move along, and in practice this is usually provided by metal wires. Metals possess a large number of free electrons, which have a high mobility. This means that if the positive pole of a battery is connected to the negative pole by means of a metal wire, then electrons will flow from the negative pole to the positive pole, where they are in a minority. If small movable positive charges existed in metals, they would have moved in the opposite direction. Such positive charges do not exist in metals, but an electrical current is still defined as if positive charges were moving. This means, in the example above, that the movement of electrons from the negative pole to the positive pole is described as an electrical current flowing from a positive pole to a negative pole.

Summarising, a flow of electric current is so defined that it always flows in an external circuit from positive to negative. This is in complete agreement with the first statement in Chapter 2, that a flow will always go from a high level to a low level, in this case from a high potential to a lower potential.

Owing to the electrochemical reactions between the battery plates and the battery acid in an accumulator, the electrons which leave the negative pole and travel through a wire to the positive pole are continually supplied internally, while the electrons arriving at the positive pole are also collected internally by an electrochemical reaction at the positive pole. For these reactions, charged particles in the battery acid are also involved, positive ones moving from the anode and negative ones from the cathode. These charged particles are called ions, and one can distinguish between negative ions and positive ions. Just as metals always possess electrons for electrical current transport, many liquids possess positive and negative ions for the transport of an electrical current.

Such liquids are called electrolytes and are usually acids, bases or liquids containing dissolved salts. All biological fluids are electrolytes: blood, for instance, contains sodium ions, potassium ions and calcium ions. What this implies for patients' safety will be discussed in Chapter 12.

It will now be obvious that if the poles of a battery, or any other voltage source, are externally connected to each other, by a metal or by an electrolyte, the result will always be the flow of an *electrical current* in the whole closed circuit. The direction of this current will be such that it flows from positive to negative in the external circuit. In metals, the transport is provided by electrons flowing in a direction opposite to the direction of the current flow; in electrolytes by positive ions moving in the same direction as the current flow, and by negative ions moving in the opposite direction.

Comparing the concepts of voltage and current, it can be seen that *current is the movement of electrical charges*, while *voltage is the tendency for charges to move, regardless of whether they really can move or not.*

The value of the current flowing round in a circuit can be measured by a current meter (see Chapter 9) connected in series with the voltage source and the rest of the external circuit. An indication of current flow can also be obtained by the series connection of an electric light bulb. If the light glows, the circuit is closed, because a current flows through the lamp, making it light up. If the circuit is broken somewhere then no current will flow and the lamp will not light up. Opening and closing a circuit can be done using a switch, which turns the light on or off.

Using more lamps, a choice can be made between a series or a parallel connection. Christmas-tree illumination is often made by connecting a number of small bulbs in series. The lamps are now sharing the total voltage of the outlet and each of the lamps lights

Fig. 3.1. A schematic representation of an accumulator. The direction of ion and electron flows are indicated.

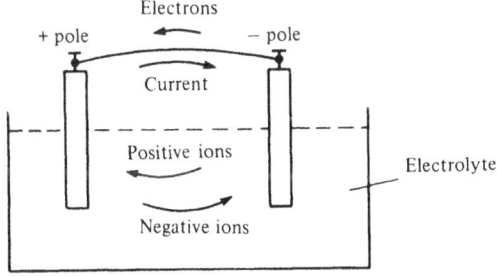

Fig. 3.2. A circuit diagram of a battery, switch and lamp.

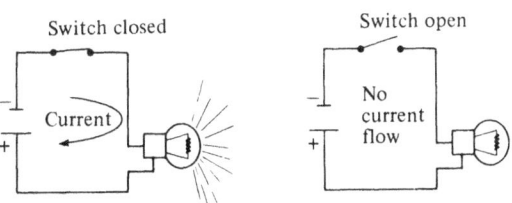

up using part of the total voltage. For instance, twenty lamps connected in series and supplied by a voltage source of 240 V will each use 12 V. A serious problem with this kind of circuit is that if one of the lamps is broken internally the circuit is no longer closed and there is no flow of current. This means that all the other lamps do not light up, which makes it difficult to find the broken bulb.

This kind of connection is therefore unsuitable for daily use for house, street and factory lighting. In these cases, use is made of the other possibility of connecting bulbs: a parallel connection. Each bulb is supplied by the main voltage and if one of the bulbs is broken, the others continue to burn. Only the total current delivered by the mains is decreased.

Direct and alternating current

In circuits in which the source is a direct voltage, the current always flows in the same direction, or in other words it is a *direct current*, often abbreviated to d.c. In the case of an alternating voltage, the current will change direction periodically; it is an *alternating current*, abbreviated to a.c. The waveform of the alternating current is the same as that of the alternating voltage source which causes the current to flow.

Direct and alternating currents are both measured in amperes, abbreviated to A, or parts of it, as mA and μA. Table 3.1 indicates the values which are met most frequently.

Fig. 3.3. A circuit diagram of a voltage source and three lamps connected in series.

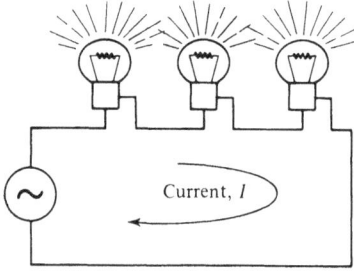

Fig. 3.4. A circuit diagram of a voltage source and three lamps connected in parallel.

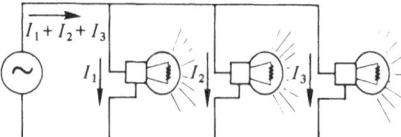

Although not explicitly mentioned previously, voltage can only serve in a circuit in which an electric apparatus is connected, as its task is to cause an electric current to flow. Any resulting action, such as light, heat, or the rotation of a motor or axle, is due to the current flow. Metal wires can be heated by current flow; if the current is high enough the metal wire will glow and can serve as a source of illumination. It is said that in this case electrical energy has been converted into other kinds of energy: heat and light.

The significance of the concept of *electrical energy* (*W*) can best be understood by the following consideration. It will be obvious that if a stone falls, the energy which the stone imparts to the earth will be larger the greater the height from which it falls. Also the energy will increase with increasing mass of the stone. The energy obtained is proportional to the mass and the difference in levels of fall. The case of electricity is quite similar. The electrical energy increases with the number of transported charged particles, which have together a total charge Q; and with the voltage, V, which causes the charge transport. Thus the following formula is obtained:

The electric energy, $W = Q V$

The total transported charge, Q, is the result of a flow of current, I, during a certain time, t. Thus:

$Q = I t$

which means that the electrical energy can also be written as:

$W = V I t$

Table 3.1. *Magnitudes of commonly occurring electric currents*

Current used by most electrical equipment	A (ampere)	1 A
Local internal circuit currents in most electronic apparatus	mA (milliampere)	10^{-3} A
Input currents of voltage-measuring devices, such as ECG recorders	μA (microampere)	10^{-6} A

Fig. 3.5. Examples of devices in which electrical energy is converted into other kinds of energy.

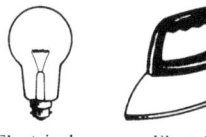

Electrical energy converted into light

Electrical energy converted into heat

The electrical energy, W, is expressed by the unit watt second, abbreviated as W sec or W s, also called a joule (J). The electrical energy necessary for defibrillating the human heart (see Chapter 11) is also expressed in W s or joules (J). On a defibrillator there is always a control marked with W s or joules by which the operator can adjust the required energy necessary for an adequate defibrillation.

Large energies are expressed in kilowatt hours, kWh, which every householder will be acquainted with because electric energy is charged per kWh. It will now be obvious that apparatus which uses larger currents is more expensive to use than low-current apparatus, and that the time the apparatus is in use is a factor in the cost of electrical energy. The energy used per unit of time, per second, is calculated by dividing the expression found for energy by t. This is called the *electric power*, represented by the letter P. Thus:

$$P = V I$$

The electric power, P, is measured in watts, abbreviated as W. Most manufacturers indicate the electric power of their products by the number of watts which the apparatus will consume. Multiplying this by the length of time the apparatus is in use gives the energy consumed by the apparatus and thus its operational cost.

Summarising, two more basic electrical concepts have now been introduced, namely electrical energy and electric power, which are directly related to the flow of electric current through an electrical apparatus.

As already mentioned, a wire through which a current flows will be heated due to the conversion of electric energy into heat. This effect is used in an electric radiator, but occurs in principle in every wire, including the wires which connect electric apparatus to the mains. These wires should not warm up, of course, because this would be dangerous. Therefore the factories which manufacture electrical apparatus provide each apparatus with a mains flex or cord and corresponding plug. The wires are sufficiently thick not to heat up significantly when the maximum current consumption of the particular apparatus occurs. This means that no cord should be used without first knowing if it is appropriate. If an electrical cord does warm up, then there must be something wrong with the cord or the apparatus, and the equipment must be switched off immediately and a technician called in.

As already mentioned, a current can also flow through electrolytes, such as battery acid, blood and infusion liquid, due to the

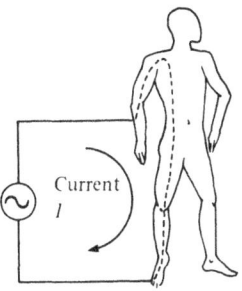

Fig. 3.6. A circuit
diagram of a voltage
source and a human
body connected to it,
resulting in a current
flow through the body.

transport of positive and negative ions in the liquid. This means
that a current will flow through the human body, if it is part of
an electrical circuit.

A current can be felt as a slight tingling if the two poles of a
4.5 V battery are placed against the tongue. Unfortunately, the
body will often complete an unsuspected circuit, allowing a current to flow. This current can be dangerous, especially if the
current flows near the heart. This is further described in Chapter
12. Here only two examples of leakage current are mentioned.

As described in Chapter 2, the potential of the earth is 0 V. If
a human being makes contact with the earth, particularly by
standing on a wet floor, then a large current will flow through his

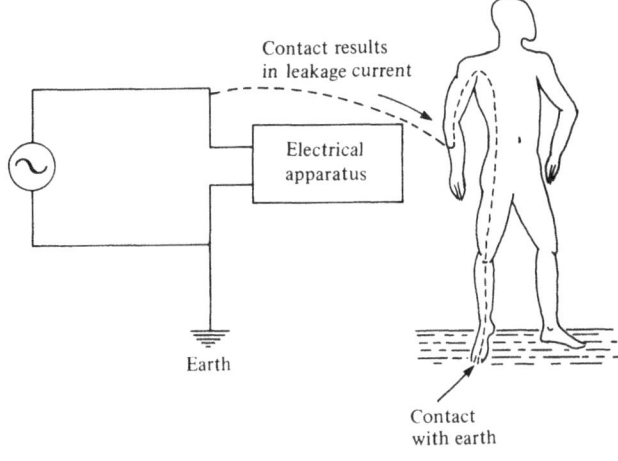

Fig. 3.7. A circuit
diagram of the mains
supply connected to
an earthed electrical
apparatus and a human
body, accidentally
connected in parallel,
resulting in a leakage
current through the
body.

Fig. 3.8. A circuit
diagram of a battery
and an electrical
apparatus which is not
earthed, which means
that no leakage current
will flow through an
earthed human body.

body to earth if he accidentally contacts a voltage which is not
0 V with respect to the earth. This situation can occur with electrical equipment with a mains supply.

Battery-supplied equipment is not usually earthed, and accidental contact by an earthed person will thus not cause a current
flow, because no circuit will be closed. Battery-operated equipment is therefore safer than equipment with a mains supply.

4. Conduction of an electric current

As seen in the previous chapter, an electrical current can only flow in a circuit which has a voltage source and is closed. This means that all parts of the circuit have to be able to transport electrical charges (electrons or ions), or in other words, all parts must have current-conducting properties. Metals are good electronic conductors and electrolytes, such as blood or sweat, are good ionic conductors.

If it is necessary to prevent a current flowing, materials which have poor conducting properties, called *insulators*, must be used. Insulators do not contain mobile electrons or ions. Good insulators include most plastic materials, ceramics, oil and air. Air is used as an insulator in most switches. When a piece of apparatus is switched off, contacts are separated mechanically; the air between the contacts is then the insulating part of the circuit, preventing the flow of any current.

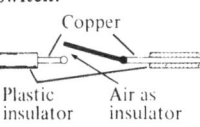

Fig. 4.1. A schematic representation of a switch.

Moisture will reduce the insulating properties of air and other insulating materials, so great care must be taken when there is moisture in the neighbourhood of electrical equipment. Plug connections which have poor watertight properties must never be used in the vicinity of a patient or in an operating theatre where liquids can easily be spilled (see Chapter 12).

Each material can be characterised and classified by its current-conducting properties. For instance, copper will conduct current more easily than iron or aluminium. This is the reason that copper is nearly always used in electrical cables. On the other hand, ceramics are better insulators than, for example, wood.

Between the materials which are good conductors and those that are good insulators, there is a class of so-called semi-conductors. These materials are used for various electronic components such as transistors (see Chapter 7).

It is obvious that there must be a relation between the value of a current in a closed circuit, the value of the voltage source in this circuit and the conducting properties of the materials which constitute the circuit. If the same voltage is applied to two circuits with different conducting properties, less current will flow through the circuit with the poorer conducting properties. If the voltage applied to an electric circuit is increased then more current will flow through that circuit.

This leads to the following equation:

$$I = V G$$

in which I is the current, V the voltage and G the conductance.

As well as the concept of electrical conductance, use is made much more frequently of the concept of *electrical resistance*, which is the reciprocal of conductance. The better a material conducts an electric current, the more easily a current will flow through it, and thus the lower is its resistance. A poor conductor corresponds to a high resistance. This can be expressed in the following equation:

$$R = \frac{1}{G}$$

in which R is the symbol for resistance.

Consequently the relation between resistance R, voltage V and current I is:

$$V = I R$$

This is known as Ohm's Law (named after G.S. Ohm). This law says that for a given resistance, R, the current flowing through it will be proportional to the voltage across it. With a fixed value of V, the current will increase with a decrease in R and vice versa: an increase in R will result in a smaller current.

The value of a resistance is measured in ohms, abbreviated with the Greek symbol Ω, or in multiples, for example kiloohm, $k\Omega = 1000\ \Omega$, and megaohm, $M\Omega = 1\,000\,000\ \Omega$.

A piece of wire, made from a certain metal, will have a certain resistance. The resistance of a long thin wire is higher than that of a short thick wire of the same metal. Resistors of various values can be made by winding wire around a ceramic tube.

Several resistors connected in series will increase the total resistance in a circuit, causing the current to decrease. The resulting resistor is the sum of the separate resistors.

Fig. 4.2. The resistance value of a resistor is determined by its dimensions.

Fig. 4.3. The current through a resistor is determined by the applied voltage and the resistance value.

Fig. 4.4. The connection of resistors in series results in a higher total resistance value.
$R = R_1 + R_2 + R_3 + R_4 + R_5$.

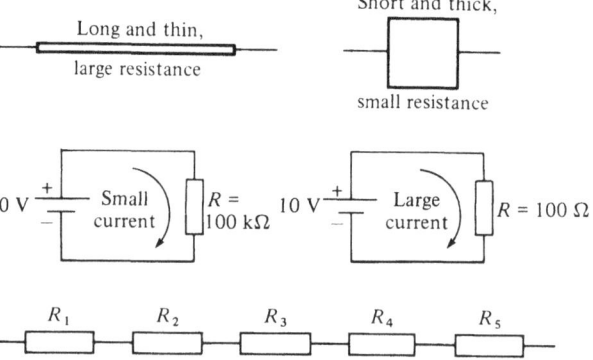

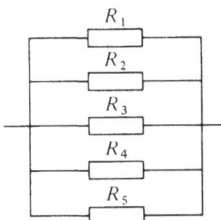

Fig. 4.5. The connection
of resistors in parallel
results in a lower total
resistance value $1/R =$
$1/R_1 + 1/R_2 + 1/R_3 +$
$1/R_4 + 1/R_5$.

On the other hand, a parallel connection of resistors will reduce the total resistance and so increase the current flowing through the circuit. The resulting resistor is the reciprocal of the sum of the reciprocals of the separate resistors.

Summarising, we conclude that resistors connected in series result in a higher resistance and thus in a lower current, while resistors connected in parallel result in a lower resistance and a higher current.

Note that these considerations are also applicable to liquids, which means that a liquid which accidentally 'shunts' a current path has the effect of a parallel connection, and thus the current automatically increases. This is the danger which is always present when liquids are spilled in the neighbourhood of electrical equipment (see Chapter 12). In this way an insulating system can be changed into a conducting one!

A special case of a resistor is an electric fire. The element is in fact a piece of wire with a relatively high resistance. Connecting the fire to a voltage source will result in a current flowing through the element; the value of this current is fixed by the values of the supplied voltage and the resistance of the element. The element must have a resistance of a value which ensures that the current will heat the element sufficiently to glow but not burn. The manufacturer therefore chooses the resistance of the element so that it will do the job over a long period of time if a limited current is passed through it.

A maximum voltage is also recommended for an indicator lamp. For example, if a lamp manufactured for 6 V is connected to a 3 V voltage source it will hardly light up. Using the same lamp connected to 6 V will provide the amount of light calculated, but connecting this lamp to 9 V will give a very bright light, but the lamp will very quickly burn out. Thus an important part of light-bulb manufacture is making elements with various resistance values.

As mentioned in the previous chapter, the power of a lamp may be indicated on it, the power being the product of the prescribed voltage and the resulting current.

Another special case of a resistor is a fuse. A fuse is a piece of wire which will melt when overheated, when a current in excess of a certain maximum flows through it. A fuse is therefore always used in series with a circuit in which a maximum value of current must not be exceeded (Fig. 4.6 a & b).

Various circuits in electrical devices may overheat if the cur-

rent passing through becomes excessive. These circuits therefore
are safeguarded by connecting a fuse designed to pass, for
instance, 250 mA in series in the circuit. This means that a current
larger than 250 mA can never flow in this circuit. Further, each
complete electrical apparatus has a central fuse to prevent the
apparatus being damaged as a result of overheating due to too-
high current consumption. Fuses are also connected in series with
various outlets in every house, factory and hospital to prevent the
cables in the walls heating up too much due to excessive current
flow.

As already described, many liquids, especially electrolytes,
conduct electrical currents – in this respect they behave like

Fig. 4.6. (a) A circuit diagram of a voltage source and an electrical apparatus in which a fuse in connected in series to protect the apparatus against excess current. (b) Examples of various types of fuses.

(a)

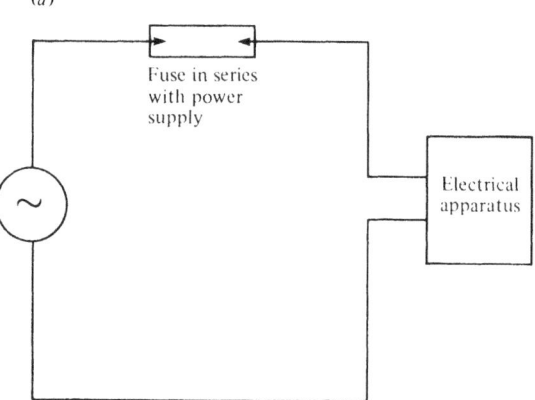

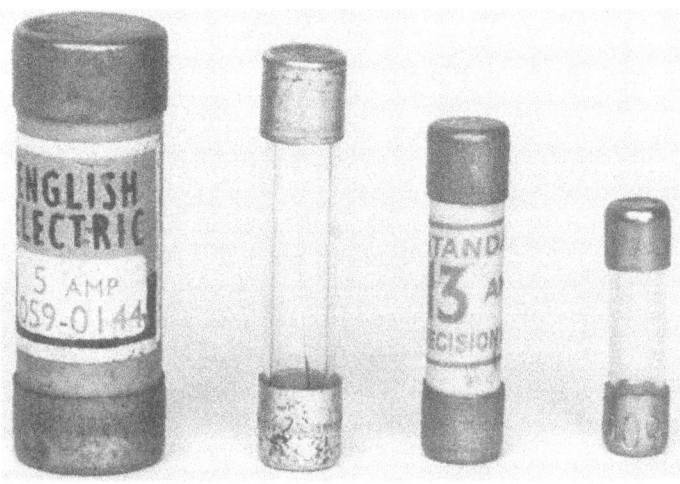

metals. A column of electrolyte, for instance a catheter filled with saline, can be considered as a resistor. The resistance of such a resistor decreases when the concentration of dissolved salts increases. A film of liquid, for instance sweat, can also be considered as a resistor. Even a thin film of sweat can have a rather small resistance across the skin because of its large area, resulting in a relatively low shunt resistance between electrodes (see Chapter 9 for consequences).

Besides the resistance of metal wires and electrolyte films, the junction between a metal and an electrolyte also behaves as a resistor. This is the case with all measurements of bioelectric events, such as ECG, EEG and EMG, where patients are connected to the instruments by metal plates, the so-called surface electrodes. In this case the resistance is called the *electrode resistance*. The value of an electrode resistance appears to be very important in various applications (see Chapter 6). One of the major prob-

Fig. 4.7. A film of sweat causes a resistive shunt between electrodes.

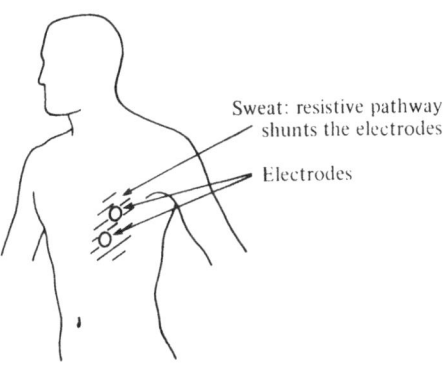

Sweat: resistive pathway shunts the electrodes

Electrodes

Fig. 4.8. The contact between an electrode and the human body behaves as a (rather complicated) resistor.

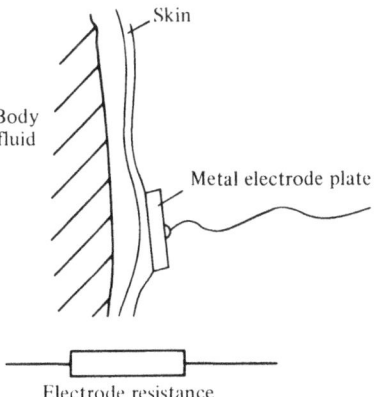

Skin

Body fluid

Metal electrode plate

Electrode resistance

lems is that a metal electrode does not make a direct contact with the internal electrolyte of the body because in most clinical cases the skin is in between. Because the skin, especially its outer layer, is rather dry and often a little greasy, the contact between electrode and body liquid is poor, presenting a high resistance if correct procedures are not followed.

These measures usually consist of cleaning the skin with alcohol, in order to remove the greasy film at the places where electrodes have to be attached, then chafing away the dry skin cells and finally soaking the skin with a 'solid electrolyte' called electrode paste, which makes the remaining skin a good ionic conductor. The result of these preparations is that the electrode resistance is considerably decreased. The effect of the various preparations separately or together is shown in Table 4.1.

As can be seen from the table, careful preparation by the user will considerably decrease the electrode resistance. The manufacturers depend upon this careful preparation when specifying the capabilities of their equipment. A poor recording of bioelectric voltages due to high electrode resistances is not the fault of the equipment, but of the user. Electrodes will be further described in Chapter 6.

Table 4.1. *The effect of pretreatments on electrode resistance*

Degreasing	Chafing	Electrode paste	Electrode resistance
x			Reduced by a factor of 60
x	x		Reduced by a factor of 250
x	x	x	Reduced by a factor of 1000

5. Various electrical components used in electromedical equipment

A large number and variety of components can be distinguished inside every piece of electronic equipment. As with biological cells, they all have a specific function and each component is connected to others to form the basic circuitry of each instrument. It is not possible, within the scope of this book, to review all the components and circuits which can be built from them, and only those which are of particular concern to the operator of the equipment will be described. In general, these are the components or functions which can be altered by controls outside the instrument, such as switches, plugs, potentiometers and adjustable filters. To explain the operation and function of these components, the principles of the resistor, capacitor and inductor have to be understood. All these concepts will be described in the following sections.

The switch

As mentioned in the previous chapter, a current can only flow in a closed circuit. The function of opening and closing a circuit is fulfilled by a switch, which can be either double poled or single poled. In the first case the circuit is connected via the switch to the voltage source by an open or closed contact at both poles of the voltage source, in the second case at only one pole.

Breaking the circuit at only one place is sufficient to block the current, but in the case of a double-pole switch the whole apparatus is completely disconnected from the voltage source. If the voltage source is the mains supply then this is an advantage for patient safety. A power switch with the indication 'on' and 'off' is an example of a double-pole switch.

Fig. 5.1. Circuit diagrams of a voltage source connected to an electrical apparatus by means of a double-pole or a single-pole switch.

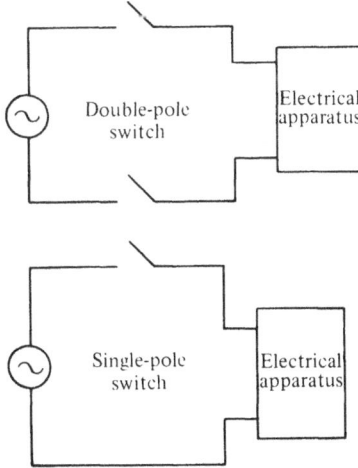

Single-pole switches are often used for opening and closing internal circuits, for instance starting or stopping a motor drive in a recorder. Rotational-step switches are often used for more complicated switching functions. In all cases these are basically the same; opening or closing two contacts. In the closed position the contacts are pressed against each other by a spring, while in the open position they are mechanically separated.

It will be clear that in the closed position the circuit may be affected by dust or grease between the contacts, and that in the open position the insulation will be far less if moisture is present between the contacts. This means that electronic equipment has to be handled carefully, implying not only proper operation of the switches, but also correct storage, cleaning and preparation of the equipment before use.

The plug

Frequently an apparatus is not continuously connected to the mains or to other equipment. The reason for this is to make the use of the equipment more flexible. The necessary connections can then be made for each specific application. These connections are provided by plugs and sockets.

There is a large variety of plugs with screw-on, snap-on and sliding connections. They all have one thing in common: two or more wires have to be connected with each other, and for this purpose the plugs contain two or more pins or holes. This means that extra care must be taken with plug connections, which are seldom watertight, in order to ensure that moisture is kept out, so as to be able to rely on the insulating properties of the materials used in the plug.

For a reliable contact between plug and socket the casings of

Fig. 5.2. Various types of single-pole and double-pole switches.

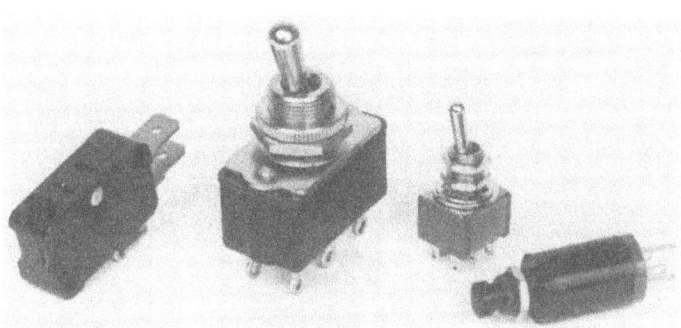

Fig. 5.3. Various types of plugs and their corresponding cables.

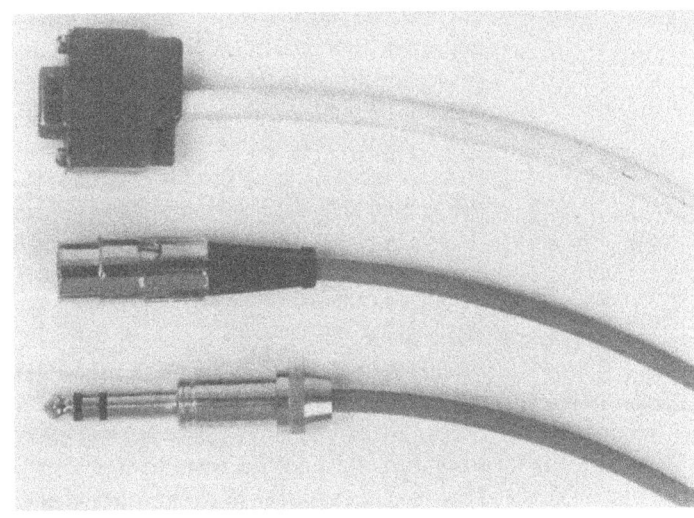

Fig. 5.4. (a) This manner of disconnecting a plug is wrong. (b) Proper disconnection of a plug, by grasping the plug case itself.

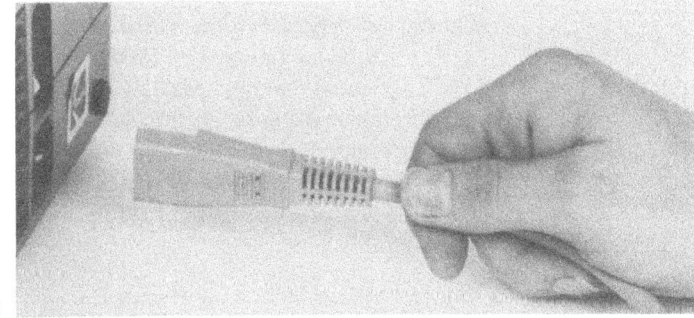

(a)

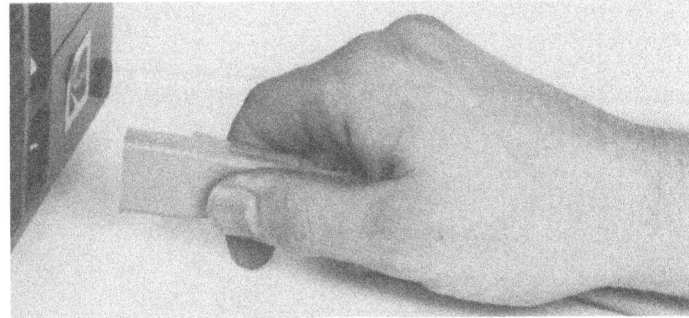

(b)

the plugs are usually tightly connected to each other. This means that when disconnecting a plug the casing itself must be grasped; a disconnection should never be made by pulling on the cable, which is only internally soldered to the plug pins.

To facilitate the use of electromedical equipment, electrode leads are often made of flexible materials. However, this makes them vulnerable, especially at the lead–plug connection.

Summarising: plug connections are essential for flexibility of use but they must be handled carefully.

The resistor

As already mentioned in the previous chapter, a resistor can be made from a wire with a certain resistivity. Nowadays, films of carbon are used in almost every type of electronic apparatus for attaining correct conditions of current flow in the internal circuits. There is a large variety of resistors in the range of 10 Ω up to 10 MΩ. The value of each specific resistor is either printed directly on to its insulating coat, or indicated by means of a colour code.

If it is required to measure the current in a closed circuit, and among the resistors in the circuit is one of a known value (R) connected in series, then the current through this resistor will develop across R a voltage $V = I \times R$ in accordance with Ohm's Law. This means that by measuring this voltage the current can easily be calculated as $I = V/R$ (V is measured and R is a known constant value).

Another example of the use of a resistor is a voltage divider, which is a way of making use of only part of the voltage of a volt-

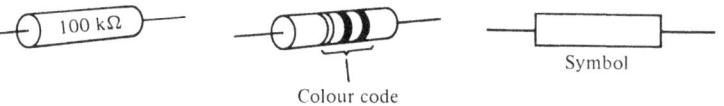

Fig. 5.5. Examples of resistors with indicated values, and their symbolic representations.

100 kΩ

Colour code

Symbol

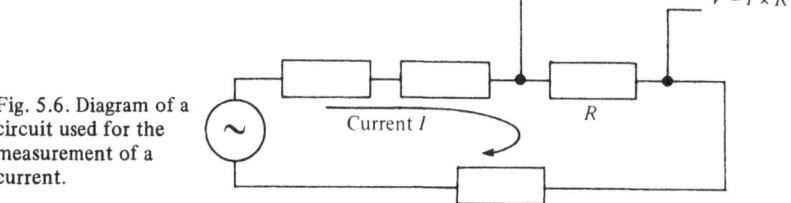

Fig. 5.6. Diagram of a circuit used for the measurement of a current.

$V = I \times R$

Current I

R

Fig. 5.7. A circuit
diagram of a voltage
divider;

$$V_{out} = \frac{R_2}{R_1 + R_2} \, V_{in}$$

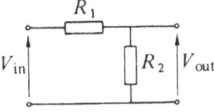

age source. If two resistors, each having the same resistance value,
are connected in series across a voltage source, then the current
through the resistors will develop half of the total voltage across
each resistor.

If the value of the resistances are in the proportion 3 : 1, for
example 3 kΩ and 1 kΩ, then the voltage across the smaller
resistance is one-quarter of the total voltage. In this way it is
possible to produce voltages smaller than the original voltage
source. This principle is used in a very flexible way in the concept
of a potentiometer, which will be described in the following
section.

The potentiometer

A potentiometer is a resistor which can be divided into two parts
by means of a sliding contact. This sliding contact can move
between the two ends of the resistor, thus creating a variable voltage divider. Usually the resistor is round, so that the sliding contact can be rotated along the resistor.

A potentiometer is mounted behind most of the rotatable
knobs on electronic equipment. Turning the knob is in fact varying resistance of the circuit and thus changing a current or a
voltage.

An example of such a control circuit is when the light intensity
of a lamp is adjusted by varying the current passing through it. If
a resistor is mounted in series with the lamp and connected to the
voltage supply, this resistor will then regulate the current in
accordance with Ohm's Law. If this series resistor is variable, then
turning the knob, and hence the sliding contact of the potentiometer, will result in varying the light intensity of the lamp.

Another example is the speed variation of a direct current electric motor. The speed is usually dependent on the value of the

Fig. 5.8. The prin-
ciples and symbol of a
potentiometer.

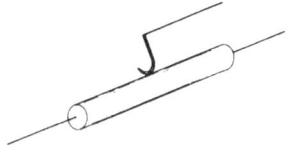

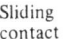

Sliding
contact

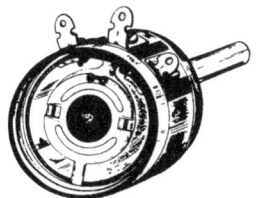

Rotating
contact

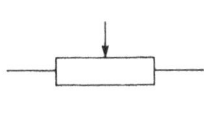

Symbol

Fig. 5.9. A circuit
diagram of adjustable
illumination.

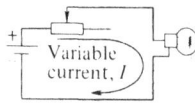

Fig. 5.10. A circuit
diagram of adjustable
motor speed.

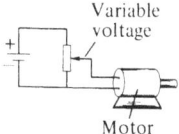

Fig. 5.11. A circuit
diagram of an electro-
magnet with adjustable
magnetic force to
attract iron filings.

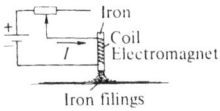

Fig. 5.12. A schematic
representation of a
relay.

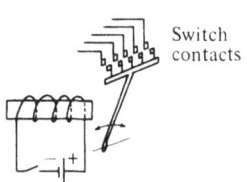

voltage supplied, so the speed of an electric motor connected to a
voltage source with a variable resistor can be controlled very
easily.

The coil

When a magnet moves with respect to a coil of conducting wire,
a voltage is produced across the ends of the coil. This is the basis
of the dynamo described in Chapter 2. If, however, a current
flows through a coil wound around an iron bar, the bar becomes
a magnet. Such a magnet is called an electromagnet, and it can
attract pieces of iron. The force of attraction can be controlled
by adjusting the current through the coil.

An oculist can use an electromagnet for removing pieces of
iron from the eye. Switches in many instruments can be opened
or closed by electromagnetic attraction. This principle of controlled switching has led to the construction of a device called a
relay. This is a switch, often a compound switch of, for instance,
ten contact pairs, in which the switching action is activated by the
attraction of the movable part of the switch by an electromagnet.
Often this electromagnet needs only a low voltage and current,
while the relay contacts can switch much higher voltages or
currents.

Another example of the application of the electromagnetic
effect is the transformer. If a coil around a bar of iron is connected
to an alternating voltage source then an alternating current will
flow through the coil. The result is that a magnetic field is induced
in the bar. This field also alternates. If a second coil is wound
around the iron bar, the alternating field produces the same result
as if a magnet placed in the position of the bar was moving. The
result is that, as in the case of a dynamo, the second coil generates an alternating voltage. This principle is called magnetic
induction. By means of this principle, it is possible to transform
an alternating voltage supplied to a primary coil into an alternating
voltage at the ends of a secondary coil. This device is called a
transformer.

A transformer can transform alternating voltages to lower or
to higher values, depending on the number of windings of the primary and secondary coils. In fact more windings can be considered
as a series connection of coils, each with one winding. Consequently the total voltage from N windings is equal to N times the
voltage from one winding.

Almost all electronic equipment designed for mains supply has a built-in transformer in order to supply the different circuits in the specific apparatus with the necessary a.c. voltages. Rectifiers can be used to convert a.c. to d.c. voltages.

If the number of effective secondary windings of a transformer can be controlled by contacting them with a sliding contact, a variable voltage source, called a voltage-variable transformer, is created, similar in principle to a potentiometer. The difference is that a voltage-variable transformer can only be used for alternating voltages, while a potentiometer operates for either a.c. or d.c. In practice, variable transformers are used for circuits which need higher current levels (above 1 A), while potentiometers are more often used for low-level currents (mA range).

The capacitor

In the second chapter, special attention was paid to the phenomenon of electric charge, especially that of the attraction of positive and negative charges. If two charged plates, with charges having opposite signs, are separated by an insulator, the charges will be mutually attracted but, because they cannot move through the insulator, they cannot neutralise each other. This means that a device consisting of two metal plates with an insulator between them can store a charge. Such a device is called a capacitor.

A capacitor can be charged by connecting the two plates to a battery. After disconnection, the capacitor stores the charge, the

Fig. 5.13. A schematic representation of a transformer.

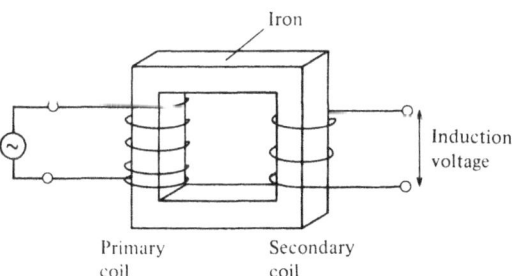

Fig. 5.14. A schematic representation of a voltage-variable transformer.

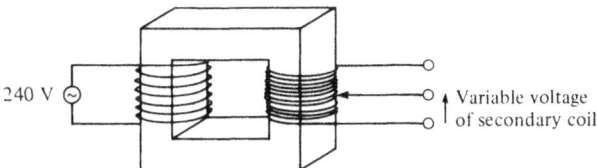

value of which depends on the dimensions of the plates, their distance apart and the properties of the insulator used to separate them. If the plates are brought in contact with each other, directly or via a resistor, the capacitor operates for a very short period as a voltage source up to the moment that the equal amount of positive and negative charges have neutralised each other. The capacitor is then discharged.

In practice, capacitors are made of two metal strips, separated by an insulating plastic layer, rolled up together and coated with an insulating lacquer.

In the same way that the resistance, R, of a resistor is expressed in ohms, the capacitance, C, of a capacitor is expressed in farads (abbreviated to F) or parts of it: for example microfarad, $\mu F = 10^{-6}$ F, nanofarad, $nF = 10^{-9}$ F, and picofarad, $pF = 10^{-12}$ F.

If a capacitor is charged by connecting it to a voltage source via a resistor, a certain time elapses before the capacitor is fully charged. Discharging the capacitor via a resistor takes the same time. This time is dependent on the values of the resistance, R, and the capacitance, C. The product RC is called the time constant of the combination, and is represented by the Greek letter tau, τ.

Charging and discharging currents have the same shape when plotted as a function of time; first a high current, which decreases rapidly (see Fig. 5.17). The reason for this shape is that during charging the additional charge necessary to further charge the capacitor to its maximum becomes smaller, since part of the

Fig. 5.15. A schematic representation and symbol of a capacitor.

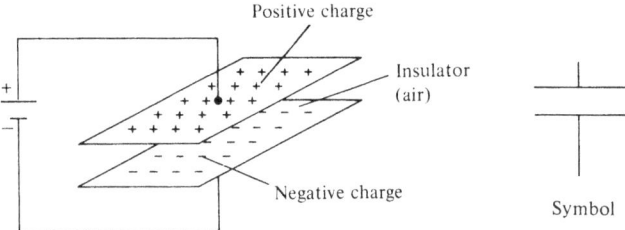

Fig. 5.16. Examples of capacitors with indicated values.

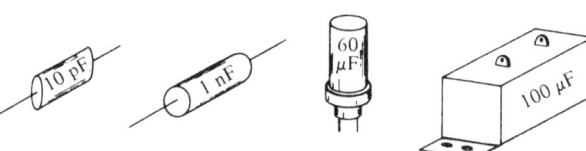

charge has already been collected on the plates. Discharging a
capacitor gives the same results; the charge flowing from the
capacitor during discharge becomes smaller the more the remaining charge diminishes.

A medical application of a capacitor is found in the defibrillator, which in fact consists of a very large capacitor which can be
charged if desired by an internal voltage source. The capacitor is
connected to the patient by means of paddles (electrodes). Pushing a switch causes the capacitor to discharge via the patient,

Fig. 5.17. (a) Charging
and discharging a
capacitor, C, via a
resistor, R. (b) Typical
charge or discharge
current curve as func-
tion of time, charac-
terised by the time
constant, $\tau = RC$.

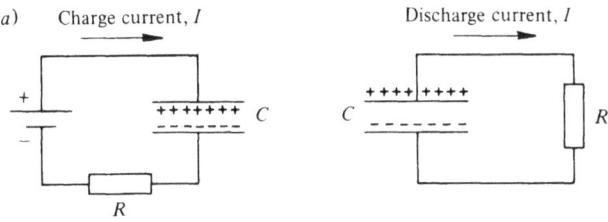

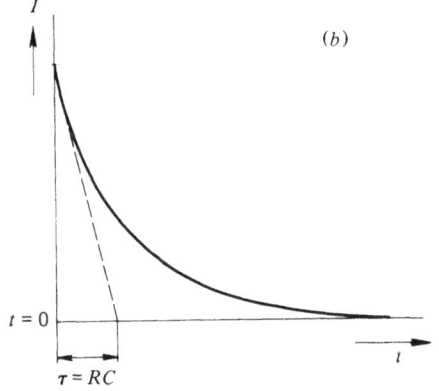

Fig. 5.18. A circuit
diagram of a defibril-
lator. A pre-charged
capacitor is discharged
via the patient.

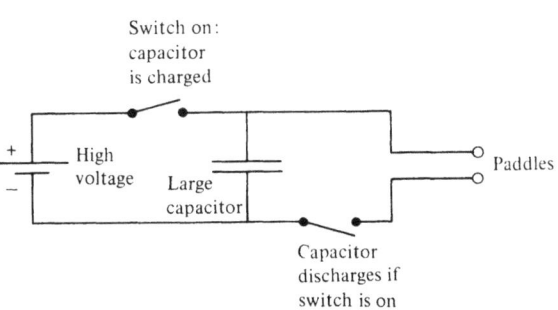

resulting in a synchronised depolarisation of the muscle fibres of the heart. This method of defibrillating from a pre-charged capacitor is convenient, because it ensures that a higher charge than that stored by the capacitor can never accidentally be delivered to the patient.

A current flowing through a patient for a fixed time, as is the case with defibrillation, corresponds to a fixed energy, this means that the defibrillator can be calibrated in watt seconds or joules (see Chapter 3).

The filter

Another important application of a capacitor is its function in a filter, which is often used in electromedical measuring equipment for suppressing unwanted artifacts in a recording.

The previous section described the charging and discharging of a capacitor connected to a d.c. source of voltage through a resistance connected in series. If the capacitor is connected to an a.c. source of voltage, the capacitor will first charge up to a positive value and when the polarity of the supply changes to negative it will charge up in the reverse direction. If the change in polarity is so rapid that the capacitor never charges up to the maximum voltage, current will flow, since charge will flow into the capacitor and never stop before it is flowing out again. This means that an alternating current will flow in the circuit, limited by the value of the capacitor and dependent on the frequency of the a.c. voltage. If the voltage is changing very quickly, the current flowing will always relate to the initial surge of current which flows when the capacitor was connected to the d.c. voltage source.

This is quite different from its behaviour in the case of direct currents, which are blocked as soon as the capacitor is charged. This different behaviour for direct and alternating currents can be used to great advantage to separate a.c. from d.c. voltages. For instance, the influence of electrode offset potentials, which are

Fig. 5.19. A capacitor blocks d.c. current, but conducts a.c. current.

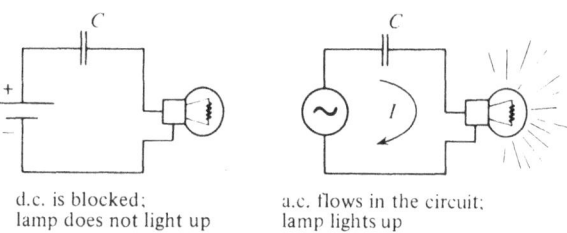

d.c. is blocked;
lamp does not light up

a.c. flows in the circuit;
lamp lights up

d.c., can be blocked by connecting a series capacitor in the electrode leads. This action is called filtering.

The effective resistance of a capacitor is a function of its
capacitance and of the frequency of the applied voltage source.
The larger the capacitance, the larger the charging and discharging
currents will be, and consequently the lower the effective resistance. Also, the higher the frequency of the voltage applied to the
capacitor, the larger the currents, and thus the lower the effective
resistance.

A frequency-dependent resistance, as the capacitor appears to
have, is called an impedance, indicated by the letter Z, and is
measured in ohms. A capacitor thus has an impedance proportional
to the reciprocal value of the capacitance and the frequency:

$$Z \propto \frac{1}{fC}$$

Note that the electrode resistance as mentioned in Chapter 4 is
also frequency dependent due to its capacitor-like properties.
Therefore it is more logical to speak of an electrode impedance
than an electrode resistance, and this will be observed in the rest
of this book.

Owing to the fact that the impedance of a capacitor is frequency
dependent, filters can be constructed that are not only useful for
separating a.c. voltages from d.c. + a.c. voltages, but also for
separating a.c. voltages of various frequencies from each other.
This result can be obtained by using a combination of a capacitor
and a resistor.

A resistor has a resistance value independent of the frequency
of an applied voltage, while a capacitor has an impedance which
decreases with increasing frequency. A voltage divider formed by
a resistor as the input of a circuit and a capacitor as the output
will thus have dividing properties which depend on the frequency
of the electric voltage. If, for a certain frequency, the impedance
of the capacitor has the same value as the resistance of the resistor,
then the voltage is equally divided between the two. The output
voltage, which is the voltage across the capacitor, is thus half of

Fig. 5.20. A capacitor
removes the d.c. com-
ponent from a com-
bination of d.c. and
a.c. voltages.

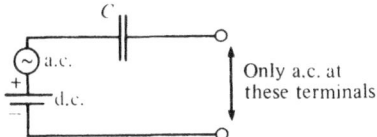

the input voltage. The higher the frequency, the less the impedance of the capacitor, and thus the lower the output voltage. The lowest frequency, which is zero frequency or in other words d.c. voltage, cannot be divided because the capacitor has an infinite impedance for d.c. The result is that lower frequencies are not attenuated by the circuit, while higher frequencies are blocked between the output and the input; this is termed 'low-pass' filtering. The frequency at which the output voltage is 0.7 times the input voltage is called the 'cut-off frequency'. It is assumed that higher frequencies than the high cut-off frequency contain no useful information about the voltage applied to the input of the filter. In the same way a filter can be constructed which blocks the low frequencies but does not attenuate the higher frequencies. In this case the input of the filter consists of a capacitor and the output of a resistor. The characteristic point of this 'high-pass' filter is again an attenuation of 0.7, which is now called the low cut-off frequency. It is assumed that lower frequencies than the low cut-off frequency contain no useful information about the

Fig. 5.21. Circuit diagram and corresponding frequency characteristic of a low-pass RC filter.

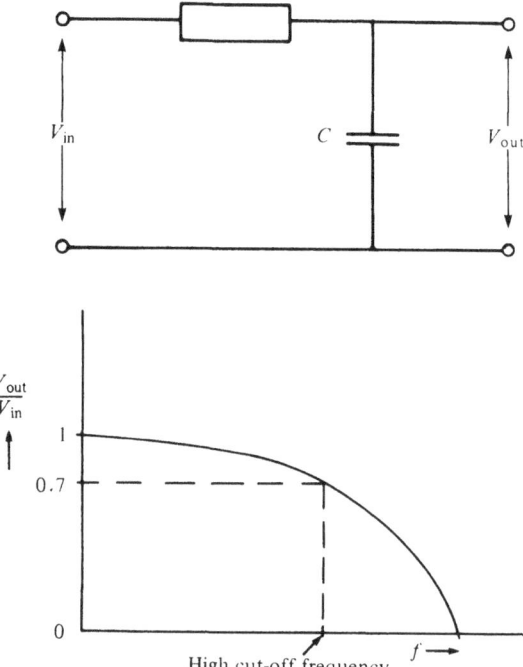

voltage applied to the input of the filter. (A low-pass filter is also called an integrator and a high-pass filter a differentiator.)

The application of both types of filters can best be illustrated by a recording in which an ECG signal and an EMG signal are mixed up. The ECG spectrum consists of low frequencies and the EMG spectrum of rather higher frequencies. If the frequency components of the ECG differ completely from the frequency components of the EMG, or in other words if the corresponding spectra do not overlap, the problem can be very easily solved.

A low-pass filter with a cut-off frequency just above the highest frequency component of an ECG would pass the ECG signal and attenuate all higher frequencies, including the EMG. Conversely a high-pass filter with a cut-off frequency just below the lowest frequency component of an EMG would let the EMG through without attenuation, but block the ECG signal.

In practice, however, the spectra of ECG and EMG are not separated, but overlap. A full ECG spectrum is between about

Fig. 5.22. Circuit diagram and corresponding frequency characteristic of a high-pass RC filter.

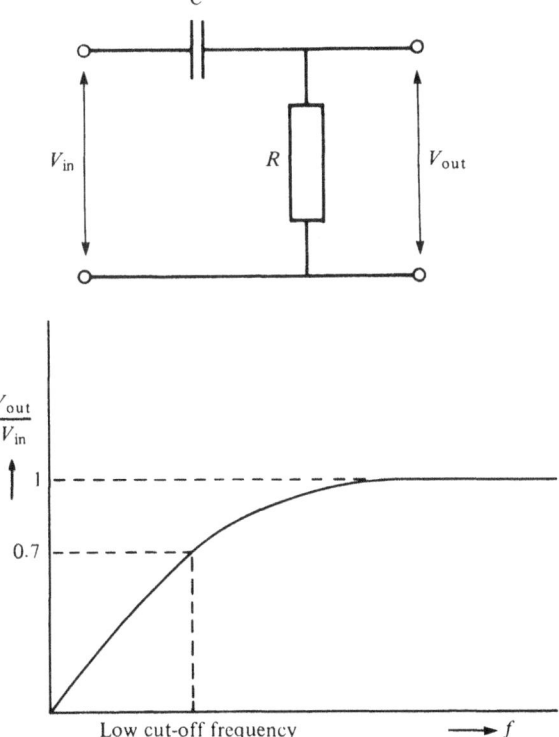

0.05 Hz and 100 Hz, while a full EMG spectrum is in the range of 20 Hz–2 kHz. This means that a compromise must be found and it will not be possible to eliminate an EMG from an ECG record-ing entirely without affecting the ECG. For instance, if a low-pass filter with a cut-off frequency of 30 Hz is used in order to cancel out almost all EMG activity, then the ECG frequency components from 30 Hz to 100 Hz are also cancelled out. This means that for the ECG the information contained in the higher-frequency com-ponents is lost, resulting in less sharp QRS-complexes and the loss of other sharp events in the ECG.

Another example of the use of a filter is in the reduction of electrode artifacts due to a variation in the electrode potentials as a result of moving electrodes. These electrode potentials are usually low-frequency signals and can thus be filtered out with a high-pass filter. Voltages in the frequency band below the low cut-off frequency of the filter are then blocked. It appears that in practical cases a low cut-off frequency of about 0.5 Hz will

Fig. 5.23. (*a*) Example of low-pass filtering for limitation of EMG activity in ECG regis-tration. (*b*) Example of high-pass filtering for limitation of ECG activity in EMG registration.

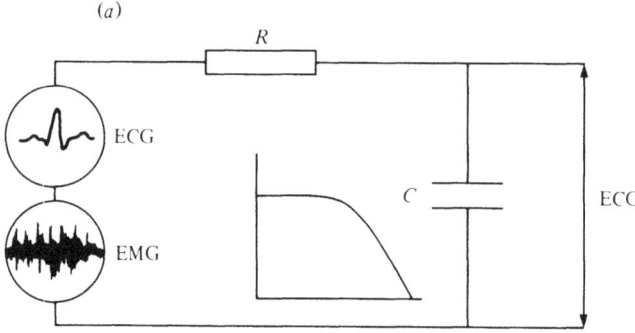

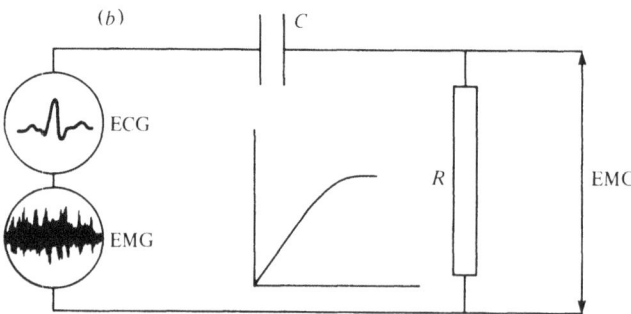

reduce the effect of electrode potentials enough to ensure a good
recording. However, it is very important to note that attenuating
the artifact also attenuates the lower frequencies of the ECG.

In general it can be stated that filters, low-pass, high-pass and
combinations of both, can be used to great advantage for reducing
artifacts in recordings. However, care has to be taken when filtering bio-electric voltages, because there is a chance that at the same
time the information which is to be obtained from the recordings
has completely or partly been removed. A warning is necessary
here: every instrument has a limited frequency pass band, so that
without the operator being aware of it, the signal is always filtered.
If additional filters are available to be switched into use for special
recordings, the position of the filter switch on the instrument
must always be noted before recording commences. More information about the practical use of filters will be given in Chapter 8,
but one more general remark about filters will be made here.

The relationship between frequency and period of a periodic
voltage has been mentioned. The period time, T, is the inverse of
the frequency: $T = 1/f$. As was explained earlier in this chapter,
an RC combination, and thus a filter, is characterised by its time
constant, $\tau = RC$ seconds. This time constant can be described in
terms of frequency. The cut-off frequency of a filter has a fixed
relation with the time constant, which is described in the equation:

$$f_{\text{cut-off}} = \frac{1}{2\pi\tau} \approx \frac{1}{6\tau}$$

This can also be written as:

$$\tau \approx \frac{1}{6f_{\text{cut-off}}}$$

This fixed relation means that filters can be described by their
characteristic time constants or their characteristic cut-off frequencies. In principle there is no difference in using the time constant, for instance 2.5 s for a high-pass filter, or using the cut-off
frequency, in this example the low cut-off frequency, which is
$1/6 \times 2.5 = 0.07$ Hz, to describe the filter properties. In electronics it is usual to describe filters by their cut-off frequencies,
e.g. 0.05 Hz−100 Hz for an ECG. In electromedical equipment
practice the concept of time constant is often used for the lowest
cut-off frequency and the concept of frequency for the highest
cut-off frequency. This leads to the description of filters by means
of a time constant and a high cut-off frequency, often indicated
on the front panels if the filters are adjustable. In the example

mentioned above the filter properties are thus indicated by $\tau = 2.5$ s and $f = 100$ Hz.

The filters which are commonly in use in electromedical measuring equipment for the registration of bio-electric voltages are listed in Table 5.1.

Table 5.1. *Filters commonly used in electromedical equipment*

Time constant (seconds)	Corresponds to a low cut-off frequency (Hz)	Often combined with a high cut-off frequency (Hz)
2.5	0.07	30
0.3	0.6	100
0.1	1.7	300
0.03	6	1000
0.01	17	—
0.003	60	—

6. Electrodes and transducers

As already described in previous chapters, the human body produces many signals, which may be physical or chemical in origin. For example, electrical signals are generated when cells such as those of the brain, nervous system and muscles are excited. Physical signals may also be detected which originate from a variety of organs, including the heart which generates sound, arms and legs which generate movements, and the body as a whole which has a certain temperature. Chemical signals may be detected in gases, indicating the concentration of various components during respiration, and in liquids such as blood and urine. All these signals may be of interest in diagnosis. However, they must be converted into a useful form for the doctor or nurse. The equipment which displays the signals is usually electronic equipment, which means that the physiological signals first have to be converted into electrical signals. The devices which fulfil this function are called transducers, of which the most commonly used types will be described in this chapter.

Electrical signals in the body are carried by ions, as already mentioned in Chapters 3 and 4, and thus have to be converted into electrical signals carried by electrons. For this purpose electrodes are used, as described in Chapter 4. As far as this chapter is concerned, electrodes are in fact a special type of transducer, used for the conversion of an electrical signal originating in the 'ionic world' into an electrical signal in the 'electronic world'. This chapter first gives a more specific and detailed description of electrodes than was given previously; afterwards other classes of transducers will be described, which convert non-electrical signals into electrical signals.

Electrodes

Most electrodes in general use are for the measurement of electrical activity of groups of cells, such as the heart, brain and skeletal muscles, resulting in the well-known ECG, EEG and EMG signals respectively. This cell-group activity is in fact the sum of the electrical activity of the individual cells and is therefore measurable at a relatively large distance from these cells, such as at the body surface. Measurements are only occasionally made at the cellular level, in which case needle electrodes have to be inserted into the tissues in order to make recordings from individual cells. This is done with brain cells, for instance, during neuro-surgery and with diagnostic measurements in neurology, where the propagation velocity of the action potentials along nerve and muscle fibres may be of interest. In medical practice, however, measurement of body-surface potentials is more common. The surface electrodes in use for this purpose will therefore be described in more detail. The behaviour of needle electrodes is similar, but in this case the observed phenomena occur at a cellular level.

The main problems with the use of surface electrodes are concerned with the electrode potential and the electrode impedance, to which reference has been made in other chapters. The electrode potential is a voltage generated between the electrode material, usually a metal, and the body tissue liquid, which is an electrolyte.

The electrode impedance is the impedance of the junction between the electrode material and the electrode gel, the value of which is mainly determined by the electrode material and the constituents of this gel. The problems with poor electrodes are that both electrode potential and electrode impedance do not have stable and constant values. This state of affairs results in additional undesirable signals, known as electrode artifacts, which disturb the signal to be recorded. Both problems can be partly solved by careful design of the electrodes, careful preparation of the skin and a stable attachment. The preparation of the skin and the effect of it has been described previously (Chapter 4). A large number of methods of electrode attachment are available, each

Fig. 6.1. EMG needle electrode used for stimulus–response experiment. Inset: concentric needle electrode.

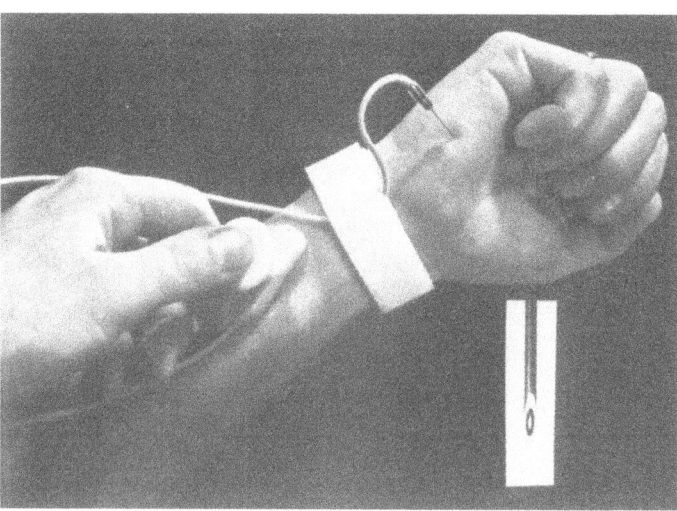

with its own specific applications and advantages or disadvantages. Easy and rapid handling plays an important part in clinical practice, and this has resulted in the development of disposable, even pre-gelled, electrodes. Personal preference as well as economic considerations influence the choice of electrodes.

Specific attention must be paid to the electrode potentials. As the voltage source must have two poles, it is logical that two electrodes should be used for any particular measurement. The bioelectric voltage to be measured is then altered by the difference in electrode potentials between the two electrodes. This potential difference, called the electrode 'offset voltage', is thus an important factor, even more so than the electrode potentials themselves. The offset voltage should, if possible, be zero and if not it must at least have a constant value, especially when low frequencies have to be measured, as in the case of ECG diagnosis. This is especially important when smaller voltages have to be measured, such as in the case of EEG recording.

Silver (Ag) electrodes which have been coated with silver chloride (AgCl) have very small and stable offset voltages. The reason is that a stable voltage is generated between the silver and the silver chloride, as in an electrochemical cell. This is also the case between the silver chloride and the electrode jelly, which is always a chloride salt. The overall electrode potential is therefore stable and fixed, resulting in very small offset voltages between a pair of silver chloride electrodes.

The silver chloride coat can easily be applied to the surface of

Fig. 6.2. Silver–silver chloride (Ag–AgCl) electrodes are preferable with respect to the stability of the electrode offset voltages.

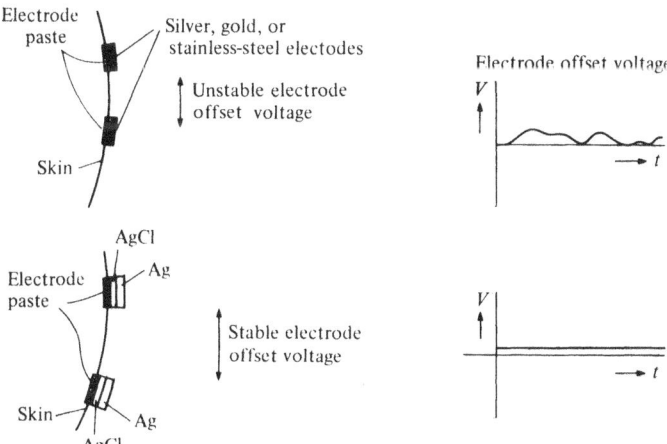

a silver disk by immersing the disk in a solution of sodium chloride and applying a voltage between the disk and a silver bar in the solution. If the silver disk is connected to the positive pole of the applied voltage, negative chloride ions will be attracted to it and precipitate on its surface. This is the most common way of coating an electrode. If the current through the disk is limited to approximately 1 mA/cm² then a stable layer of silver chloride will be deposited on the silver surface after about one hour. This layer of silver chloride, however, is very easily scratched and when it is damaged the stability of the offset voltage between a pair of electrodes is lost, usually resulting in an unstable and relatively high electrode offset voltage, often disturbing a measurement completely. Thus silver—silver chloride electrodes have to be handled carefully. They are, however, used routinely for ECG monitoring in the coronary care units of most hospitals.

Another effect with silver—silver chloride electrodes is that the chloriding process appears to result in rather low electrode impedances, which is always an advantage. The capacitor effect, that is the charge-storing capability of the electrode, is poor for a silver—silver chloride electrode, which is another advantage because it means that any disturbance of the offset voltage due to external causes, such as electrode movement or a defibrillation pulse, very quickly disappears.

With measurements where lower-frequency components are not important, as in heart-rate monitoring, or do not exist, as in the case of EMG recording, silver—silver chloride electrodes need not be used. In these cases the effects of unstable electrode offset voltages may be cancelled out or suppressed by the use of filters.

Transducers

As mentioned above, non-electrical signals from the body have to be converted into electrical signals. This must be done in order to provide the electronic equipment with signals which are related to the original physiological signals such as temperature, sound, pressure, flow or concentration.

It should be noted, however, that this is only the case if electronic recording or display is necessary. For incidental measurement of certain body signals, non-electrical equipment can be used; for instance a mercury thermometer for the measurement of body temperature. In this case, there is still the need to convert a physiological signal into a visible signal, which can be easily interpreted by the user of the measuring instrument. With a thermometer, temperature is converted into the length of a column of mercury and this length is directly calibrated in terms of temperature. Electronic equipment is necessary for continuous observation of such signals, consequently electrical transducers have to be used. The output signal of such a transducer is an electrical voltage, current or impedance, from which the value can, as in the case of the thermometer, be directly calibrated in terms of the original input signal. If the relation between the input signal and the output signal is fixed, independent of time and environmental conditions, this calibration can be done by the factory which manufactures the specific transducer. If the input—output relationship can change during use then the transducer calibration has to be carried out by the user at intervals during use, especially just before recording a measurement with the transducer. Unfortunately, many types of transducer need regular calibration, which is a disadvantage.

In general, two types of transducers can be distinguished, namely those which provide the user directly with a voltage and those which do so indirectly. The second type consists in most cases of a resistor, the resistance of which is dependent on the signal to be measured. This type of transducer requires a voltage supply in order that use can be made of Ohm's Law to calculate the resistance from the measured current resulting from the applied voltage. Safety requirements for such transducers must be high, especially if they are to be used inside the body.

The transducers most commonly in use are described below under the two classes defined above.

Transducers which generate a voltage directly

The thermocouple. A potential is generated when two different materials, in intimate contact with each other, have different temperatures at the junctions. The value of this potential varies with the temperature difference, and is especially pronounced with iron—constantan junctions. This transducer is called a thermocouple and is frequently used for the measurement of relatively high temperatures such as might be encountered in sterilisers and autoclaves. The accuracy of this transducer is not good enough for the measurement of body temperatures unless special measures are taken.

The crystal microphone. Some crystals of piezoelectric material have the property of being able to generate a voltage between their ends if pressure is applied to them. This effect is put to use in some types of displacement transducers, the crystal pick-up element of a record player being a well-known example. The crystal can also be connected to a membrane which can pick up sounds from the air. This is the principle of the crystal micro-phone, which converts sound directly into a voltage.

This type of microphone, which may be used to convert heart sounds into a corresponding voltage waveform, is used in phono-cardiography. A difficulty with this technique is that the mem-brane of the microphone can be caused to vibrate by other sounds both inside and outside the body, or by movement of the microphone itself. In other words, the microphone does not selectively detect heart sounds and the recording is therefore often disturbed by other sound artifacts. It is often the case that a conventional stethoscope provides the user with a more useful signal, mainly because one is able to listen selectively. An elec-

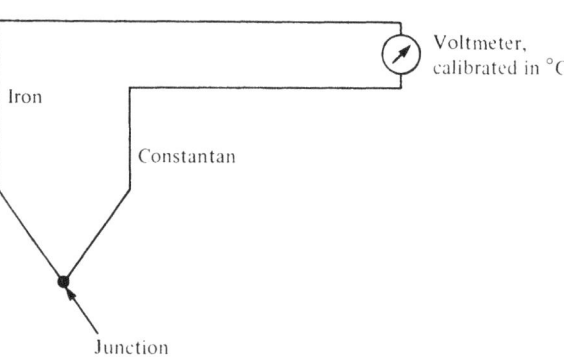

Fig. 6.3. The principle of the thermocouple for the measurement of temperature.

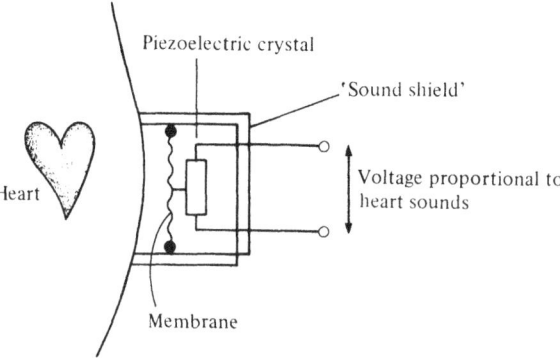

Fig. 6.4. A schematic representation of a microphone for the measurement of heart sounds (phonocardio-graphy).

tronic stethoscope based on a microphone with electronic amplifier and earphone is, therefore, an example of electromedical
equipment which may not be preferable to non-electronic equipment. Non-electronic equipment does not provide a permanent
record, however, and the electronic transducer has to be used
where a recording is needed. Artifacts have to be reduced by careful positioning of the microphone, by avoiding noisy rooms and
by filtering the output signal of the transducer.

The pH electrode. Another example of a transducer which generates a voltage directly as a function of a non-electrical input is the
pH electrode, used for measurements of hydrogen ion concentration in blood, gastric juice and other body fluids. In principle,
the pH electrode is nothing more than a thin-walled bulb of special
glass, fused to a more rigid glass tube and filled with an electrolyte. The thin glass membrane selectively absorbs hydrogen ions,
resulting in the development of a potential at the outer glass surface. The value of this potential has a fixed relationship to the
concentration of hydrogen ions in the liquid in which the electrode
is immersed. This concentration is conveniently expressed in pH
units.

The voltage across the glass membrane, which is a function of
pH, has to be measured with two electrodes, one in the solution
inside the glass bulb and one in the solution of which the pH has
to be measured. These two electrodes also generate a voltage,
which is in series with the pH-sensitive voltage across the glass
membrane. The electrodes, therefore, must be made in such a way
that they generate a constant voltage, independent of pH. The use
of silver—silver chloride electrodes can satisfy this requirement, as
explained in the first section of this chapter. As with other transducers, the pH electrode has to be calibrated, in this case with

Fig. 6.5. A schematic
representation of a pH
electrode.

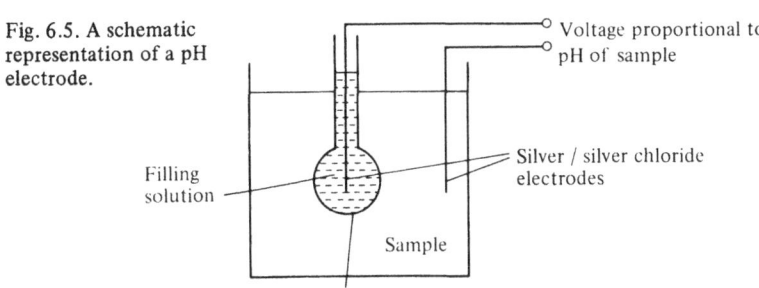

Voltage proportional to
pH of sample

Silver / silver chloride
electrodes

Filling
solution

Sample

Glass membrane

solutions of known pH. The pH of blood is normally about 7.15 and deviations from this indicate that the patient has a problem maintaining his internal acid base balance. As small changes in pH are important, the accuracy and reliability of the measurement must be good. Small pH electrodes for intravascular measurement are not as stable as larger pH electrodes. Blood pH is therefore often measured by means of larger electrodes using samples of blood taken to the apparatus remote from the patient.

A modification of the pH glass electrode can be made by the use of other types of glass, which are, for instance, selectively sensitive to sodium or potassium ions. Additional membranes can also be used to transform the electrode into a transducer for CO_2, in blood-gas measurements.

It is interesting to note that the human body itself is full of the type of transducer just described, in the form of sense organs. These biological transducers convert, mostly very selectively, all kinds of physical or chemical signals into electrical signals which are then carried along sensory nerves to the brain.

Transducers which need a voltage supply

Transducers which consist of a resistor the resistance of which is a function of an external condition, such as temperature or pressure, are used in a circuit in which the current through the transducer can be measured as a function of that parameter. This may be done by means of a series resistor, the voltage across which is, according to Ohm's Law, proportional to the current. With a constant voltage applied across transducer and series resistor, this current is inversely proportional to the transducer resistance value. The output voltage of the transducer circuit thus bears a fixed relationship to the transducer resistance and can be directly calibrated in units of the input signal. In fact, the whole circuit can be seen as a voltage divider, controlled by the external signal.

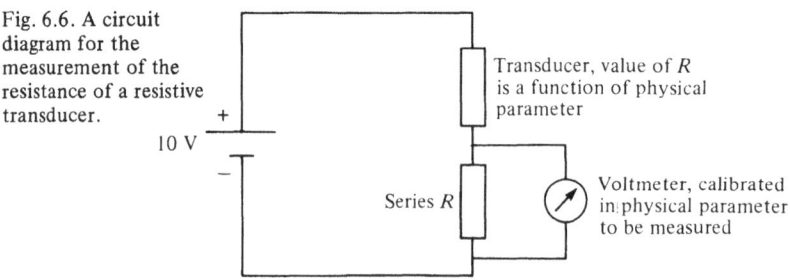

Fig. 6.6. A circuit diagram for the measurement of the resistance of a resistive transducer.

10 V

Transducer, value of R is a function of physical parameter

Series R

Voltmeter, calibrated in physical parameter to be measured

In most cases a supply voltage of the order of several volts is used in order to provide the desired accuracy. With internal measurements the insulation of the transducer wires has to be extremely good and this type of transducer has to be handled with extreme care.

In order to increase the accuracy of these transducers more sophisticated electronic circuitry is used. One of the circuits most commonly used is the bridge circuit, in which the transducer voltage divider is compared with a voltage divider consisting of fixed resistors.

The transducers of the class described in this section can be classified under three types, namely resistance as a function of temperature, pressure and light. The first two are used directly for the measurement of temperature and pressure in the human body, while the third type is used indirectly, e.g. to detect the light-transmitting properties of biological tissues. The first two transducers can also be used indirectly, for instance in cases where a stream of air or liquid changes the temperature or pressure.

Temperature transducers and related measurements. The temperature-sensitive resistor is called a thermistor. Its dimensions can be as small as one or two millimetres and therefore thermistors are very useful for mounting in the tips of catheters. A large range of thermistor probes is commercially available, for different applications, for instance the measurement of body temperature using an electronic thermometer.

An example of the thermistor being used indirectly is in the monitoring of respiration. A thermistor placed in the outer nasal passage will detect the temperature difference between cool inspired air and warm expired air. In this way a temperature

Fig. 6.7. A circuit diagram of a so-called bridge configuration.

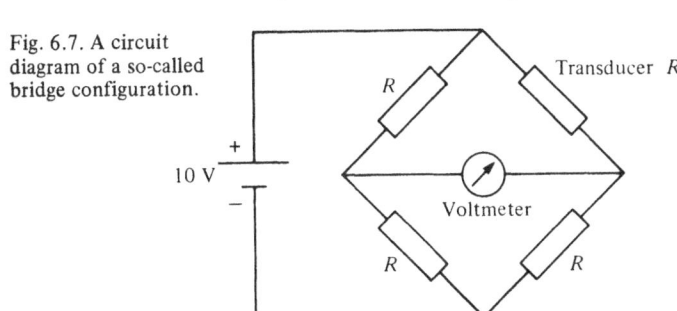

measurement can indirectly provide a measurement of respiration rate. The power supply to such a thermistor should be current-limited to prevent it from becoming warm and causing the patient discomfort.

The sensitivity of such a system may be increased by increasing the current through the thermistor in order to raise its temperature (see Chapter 3) to just above body temperature. The thermistor will now be cooled by both the inspired and the expired air. The resulting signal, measured as a change in the resistance, can thus be made more sensitive to low flow rates. The recording of the output is called a pneumogram. A rate of 12 to 18 breaths per minute is normal. The system may be used in intensive care units to indicate respiratory rates; it gives no information about tidal volume, only about respiratory activity.

The same principle of airflow detection by means of a heated thermistor is used for the detection of apnoea in neonates. For this purpose, a mattress consisting of many compartments intercon-

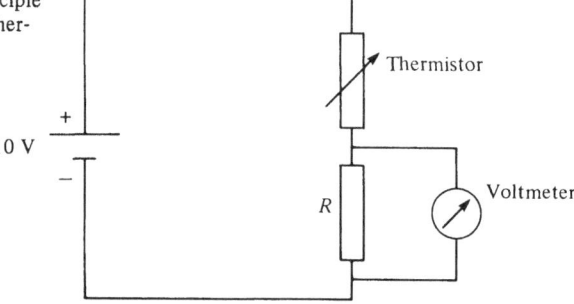

Fig. 6.8. The principle of an electronic thermometer.

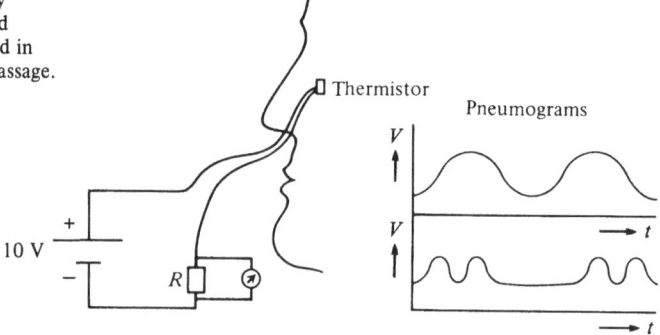

Fig. 6.9. Monitoring of the respiration by means of a heated thermistor, placed in the outer nasal passage.

nected by means of small tubes has been developed. The tubes are connected to each other via a manifold in which a heated thermistor is placed. Every movement of the neonate will cause a flow of air from one compartment to the other, resulting in a change of the resistance of the thermistor. Even respiratory movement will cause a signal. The detection system is usually constructed in such a way that an alarm signal will be switched on when no signal has been received from the transducer after a predetermined time interval.

Pressure transducers and related measurements. Pressure-sensitive transducers, under the classification of resistance change as a function of pressure or strain, have many different forms, the most simple form of which is an elastic tube filled with mercury. Contacts are made with the mercury at both ends of the tube and consequently a resistance can be measured between the two ends. It will be obvious that a variation in length of the tube will result in a longer and thinner column of mercury, thus increasing its resistance. Such a strain-sensitive transducer is called a strain gauge.

Information about respiration can be obtained by measuring the volume variations of the thorax caused by breathing, by fitting a band fitted with a strain gauge carefully around the chest. This method is not used for intensive care, because thoracic movements do not necessarily correlate with adequate ventilation.

Fig. 6.10. Monitoring of movement by detecting airflow along a heated thermistor.

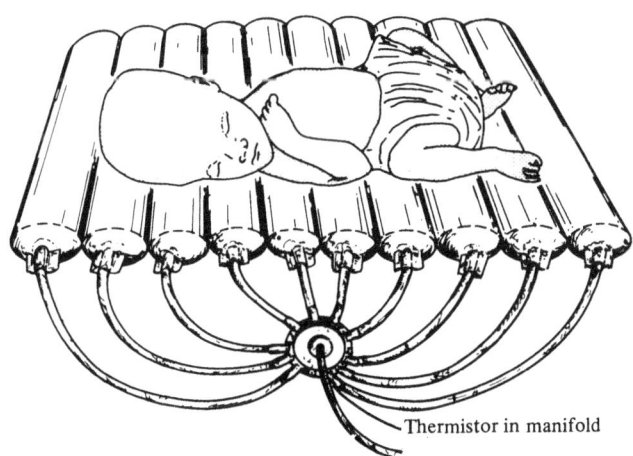

Thermistor in manifold

The volume variation of a finger or another extremity can also be measured in this way, giving an indication of the blood flow through it. This kind of measurement is called plethysmography. Another common method for plethysmography makes use of the light-transmitting properties of extremities and will be described later.

In addition to the simple strain gauges mentioned above, very small pieces of special materials, called semiconducting material, can be used as strain gauges. Often these small strain gauges are mounted on an elastic spring or diaphragm. If such a diaphragm is then mounted at the end of a tube, a pressure transducer which can measure the pressure of a liquid in the tube is produced. This type of pressure transducer is in use in daily practice for measuring blood pressures. In this case the tube is called a catheter and is connected to a needle, which is inserted into the circulatory system. The catheter is completely filled with physiological saline and often continuously flushed with a very small flow of saline to stop clotting on the needle. The pressure changes at the needle are transmitted through the filling solution in the catheter to the diaphragm, where the pressure is measured.

If the open end of the catheter is inserted into the heart, cardiac defects, such as incompetent or stenosed valves, can be investigated. This procedure is called 'cardiac catheterisation'.

The pressure transducer, consisting of a diaphragm attached to a strain gauge, has to be calibrated with respect to the atmospheric pressure. This may be done by applying the pressure of a column

Fig. 6.11. Strain gauge fitted in a band which can be attached around the chest.

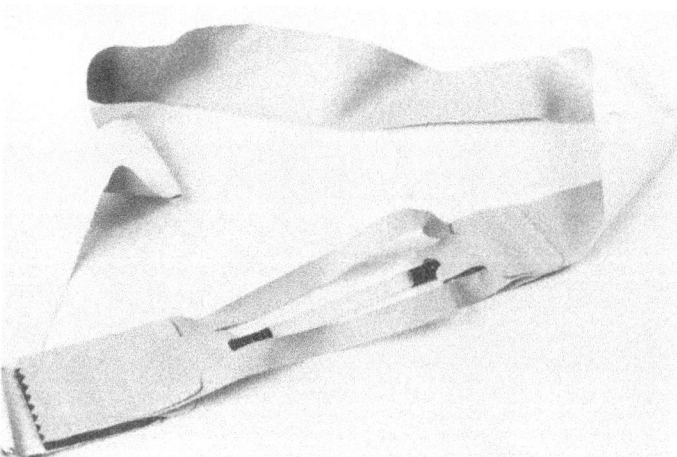

of mercury to the transducer via a tap connected in series with the catheter. The electrical output can thus be calibrated directly in millimetres of mercury.

It will be obvious that a direct connection with the bloodstream of a patient, via a highly-conducting column of saline, requires meticulous care to ensure the patient's safety. The internal insulation of the transducer has to be good and should be tested at regular intervals.

Because the actual sensing element, a strain gauge, or more often two or four strain gauges in a bridge configuration, can be compactly constructed, catheter-tip transducers have also been produced.

In this case the pressure transducer is directly mounted at the tip of a standard catheter, and no filling solution is necessary.

Fig. 6.12. External pressure transducer for connection to a catheter.

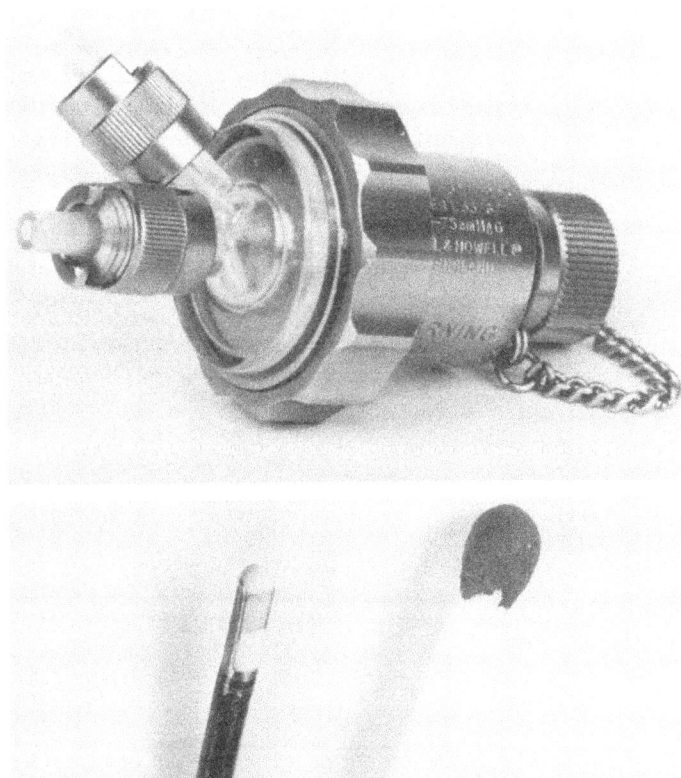

Fig. 6.13. Photograph of the tip of a catheter-tip pressure transducer.

Safety requirements, however, are now more critical, and because calibration can now only be done before and not during measurement, problems of stability and consistency of performance arise. The direct blood-pressure measurements described above provide the cardiologist with absolute values of blood pressures.

Another example of the application of strain gauges is found in an accelerometer, used for measuring the movement of extremities, for instance hand tremor. In this case the strain gauge is mounted on a strip of steel and a small weight is mounted at the end of the blade. Movement of the complete construction results in a bending of the steel, with a corresponding change in the resistance of the strain gauge. A very simple tremor transducer can thus be constructed.

Phototransducers and related devices

As mentioned previously, the conductance of some materials changes with the amount of light striking them. Using these materials, light-sensitive resistors, called photocells, can be constructed. These photocells are not suitable for direct measurements of biosignals, simply because no biological light sources exist in the human body. Photocells, however, can be used in transducers which themselves incorporate a light source. If biological tissue is placed between this source and the light-sensitive resistor, the light-transmitting properties of this tissue can be measured.

Fig. 6.14. Open view of a tremor transducer, consisting of a piece of silicon (semiconductor strain gauge) on a gold-plated plastic bar with a small weight at the end.

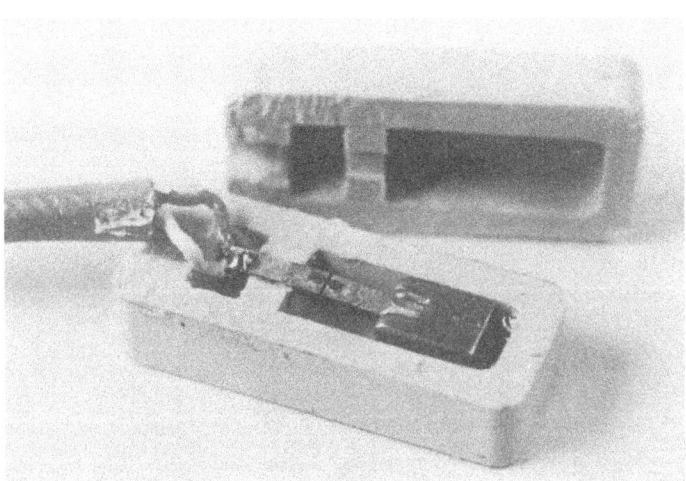

If the light source is completely screened, the light-sensitive resistor will show a resistance value as if it were in the dark, while the resistance will decrease if the screening is less. This means that blood pulsating through the tissue and so periodically changing the amount of blood in the tissue will result in a varying screening of the light source. The resistance of the photocell will consequently be changed in a like manner and will give an indication of the blood flow. It should be noted that the signals can only be interpreted relatively and that no absolute values are provided.

This type of measurement is called photo-plethysmography and is very commonly used in clinical practice, where a finger or an earlobe is often used. When a finger is used, the internal bone can screen the light source completely, so that in this case the light source and the photocell are usually placed on the same side of the finger, in which case the reflection of light by the blood is detected.

This type of transducer is usually called a peripheral pulse transducer, or in short, a pulse sensor, and is mostly used for detecting the pulse rate. Although only an indication is obtained of whether the peripheral blood flow is present or not, it is of course an important application.

An advantage when measuring heart rate by this method is that no electrical contact is made with the patient, unlike the measurement of an ECG, where electrodes are used. For safety reasons a

Fig. 6.15. Optical sensor for earlobe attachment. Note the lighted lamp on one side of the sensor and the photoresistor on the opposite side.

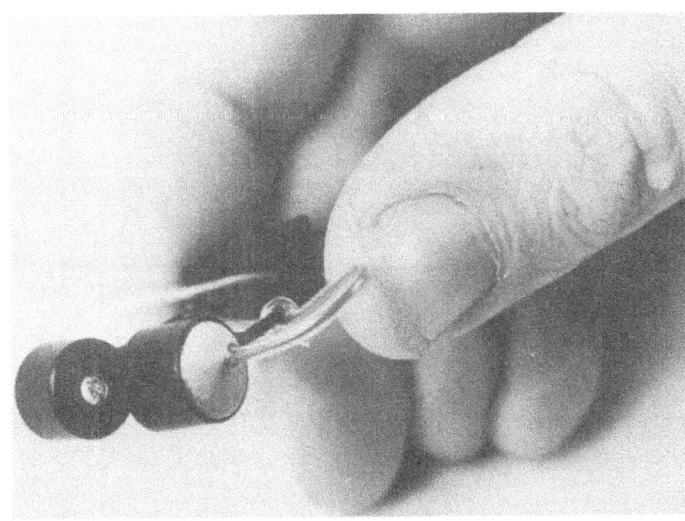

measurement which does not require electrical contact is preferable.

A serious problem with this type of transducer is that the photocell also reacts to other light sources, which may interfere with the modulated light due to the pulse. This is often a troublesome source of artifacts, giving rise to false alarms. These artifacts can be reduced by using black tape to cover the whole transducer including the tissue, but in practice this may not be convenient. Some manufacturers have solved the problem by using photocells which are not sensitive to visible light but to infrared radiation, in combination, of course, with a source which emits this type of radiation. There still remains the problem that movement of the transducer may cause a change in the volume of the tissue between the light source and the photocell, resulting in a change of the light transmission or reflection, with a corresponding change in the output of the photocell. Attempts have been made to limit this disadvantage by using specially constructed transducers.

All the transducers described up to now have been of the type based on a direct or indirect variation of resistance controlled by a physiological phenomenon. In addition to this class of transducer, other types are in use, one of which will be described here

Fig. 6.16. (a) Two examples of fingertip peripheral pulse sensors. The lamp and the photo resistor can easily be seen in the one on the left. (b) Registration of peripheral blood flow with one of the transducers of Fig. 6.15 or 6.16a.

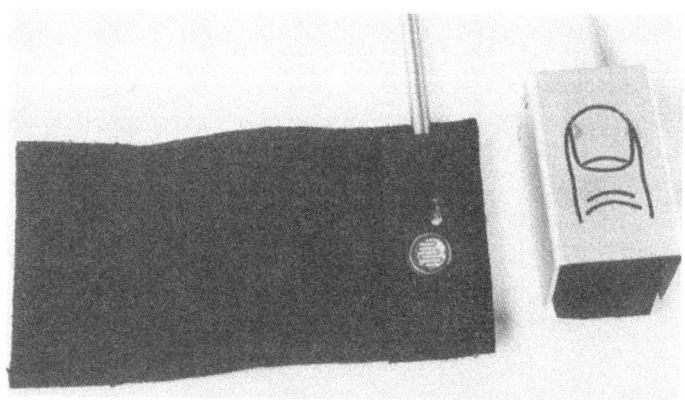

(a)

(b)

since it completes the range of effects to be mentioned. As well as the measurement of blood flow and blood pressure, blood velocity is also of importance; however, the measurement of this presents practical problems. Two methods have been developed, an electro-magnetic method and a method which makes use of ultrasound, each with its own advantages and disadvantages.

The principle of the electromagnetic blood-velocity transducer has already been described in Chapter 2, where it was explained that if a conducting wire is moved through a magnetic field a voltage can be measured between the ends of the wire (the prin-ciple of the dynamo). Because blood is a conductor, if it flows through a magnetic field a voltage can be measured across the moving bloodstream. The voltage can be measured across the blood vessel walls by means of tiny electrodes.

The transducers used induce a magnetic field in the blood-stream and contain a pair of voltage-measuring electrodes. The voltage measured between these electrodes has a pulsatile form, while the amplitude of the signal is proportional to the blood velocity. The transducer has to be brought into close contact with the blood vessel, which means that this method can only be used intracorporeally.

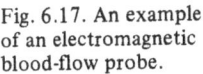

Fig. 6.17. An example of an electromagnetic blood-flow probe.

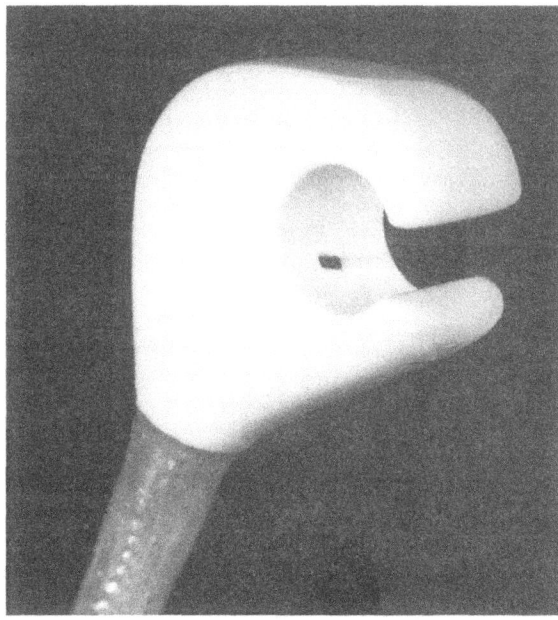

Fig. 6.18. (*a*) An ultrasound transducer used
for measuring blood
flow in the right
carotis communis.
(*b*) Corresponding
registration.

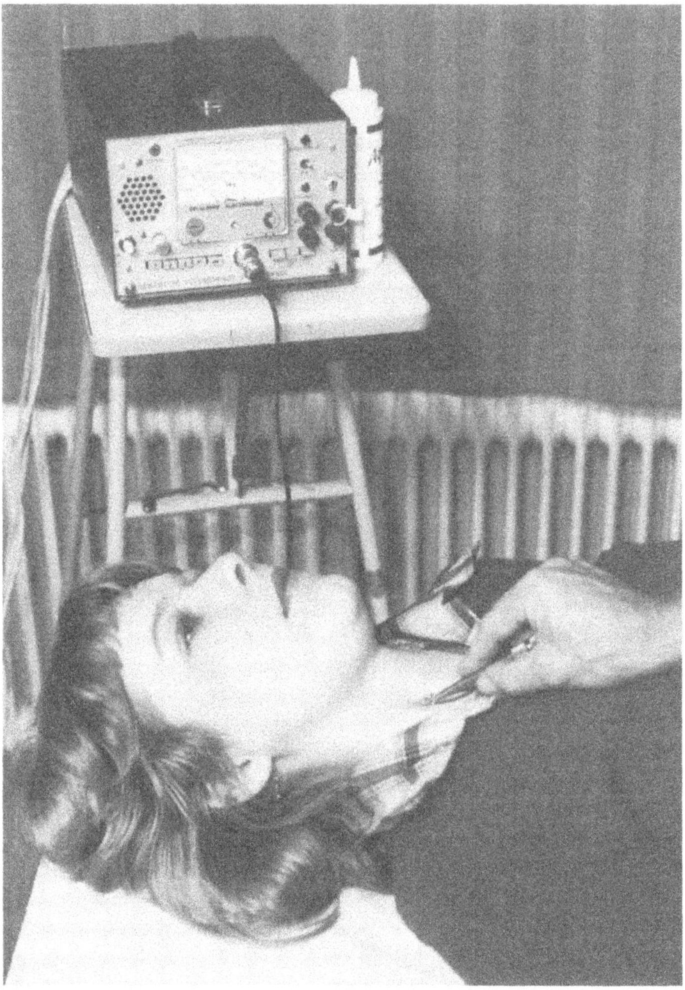

(*a*)

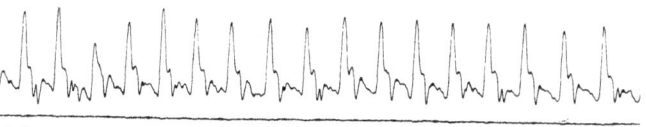

(*b*)

The other method makes use of ultrasound, the frequency of which is far beyond that of audible sounds, of the order of several megahertz. It can be generated and detected by special crystals. Ultrasound energy is propagated by biological tissue and reflected by more dense tissue. This means that the ultrasound transducer can be used externally against the skin, making contact by means of a special oil, and will receive and detect reflections from internal tissue complexes.

Using this technique all kinds of movements can be detected, not only the movement of the heart walls and valves, but also of the blood itself. From this signal, the blood velocity in a particular vessel can be calculated.

Ultrasound offers in principle an excellent way of collecting information from internal organs. The development of this equipment is now proceeding rapidly and further progress is expected in the near future.

To conclude this chapter about electrodes and transducers with examples of some of the special types, perhaps it should be stated that the use of a particular type of electrode or transducer is often a question of personal preference. No general rule can be made for recommending the types of electrodes and transducers for any particular case, and the user must build up his own experience as to which type is most suitable for the conditions under which he is attempting to make observations.

7. Electronic amplifiers

The human body contains many sources of electric potential, often picked up directly by means of electrodes, and many transducers for converting the activity of non-electrical sources into electrical signals have been described. The result is that a wide range of voltages are measured, directly or indirectly, and can be used for diagnoses. One thing that all these electrical voltages have in common is that their amplitudes are rather small, being of the order of 1 μV up to 10 mV. These values are usually too small to register on equipment like chart recorders, magnetic tape recorders or displays (see Chapter 9). It is therefore necessary to increase these small voltages to higher values, of the order of volts, and to do this electronic amplifiers have been developed. An electronic amplifier amplifies input voltages in a certain frequency band to higher output voltages. For example a 1 mV ECG voltage picked up by two electrodes and connected to an amplifier with an amplification factor (often called a gain) of 1000, appears at the output of the amplifier as a voltage of 1 V. In addition, this 1 V voltage source may be able to deliver enough current to drive, for instance, the pen motor of a paper recorder. It is not possible to

Fig. 7.1. A typical example of a biomedical amplifier plug-in unit. The low-frequency cut-off, which is adjustable by means of push-buttons, is designated with time constant values, given in seconds (s), while the high-frequency cut-off is given in the unit Hz. The amplification or sensitivity can be adjusted by a factor of 2000, while the d.c. level (offset voltage) can be shifted + or − 200 mV. In addition, a calibration pulse can be generated.

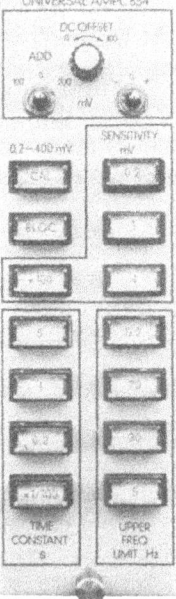

draw this current directly from the original voltage source – the actual ECG; thus in addition to amplifying the input voltage, an amplifier increases the power of the source.

An amplifier is represented schematically by means of a triangle with input and output leads. The letter A is used to represent the internal gain, which may be fixed or adjusted manually by means of a potentiometer. This front-panel control may be designated 'gain', 'size', 'amplitude' or 'sensitivity'.

The gain of an amplifier has to be such that no distortion in the output can occur. If there is a large gain, the output signal may show flat parts due to the signal level exceeding the output voltage limit of the amplifier in use.

Another important characteristic of an amplifier is the band of frequencies it passes. As described in Chapter 5, every electronic system has a limited frequency band, often set to fixed values of low and high cut-off frequencies or externally adjustable by means of built-in filters. Using an amplifier with an inadequate frequency characteristic will result in distortion of the amplified signal, as extensively described in Chapter 3.

Although it is not the aim of this book to describe the internal circuitry of electromedical equipment, it may be useful to describe very briefly some of the internal circuitry of an amplifier. Besides the passive components such as resistors, capacitors and inductors, an amplifier always contains one or more active components which do the job of amplification. As the passive components have already been described in Chapter 5, here the active components most commonly in use are described – the electronic valve or vacuum tube, and the transistor.

The active component in the first amplifiers was the electronic valve or vacuum tube, resembling an ordinary light bulb but with some additional plates and grids inside, and consequently more internal connections. Although the invention of the electronic valve made it possible to build electronic amplifiers for the first time, nowadays they are hardly ever found inside electromedical instruments because the electronic valve has been completely replaced by the transistor. In fact, the function of a transistor is similar to that of the valve but its appearance is quite different.

Fig. 7.2. An example of overflow distortion: for the right-hand part of the registration the amplification factor was tripled.

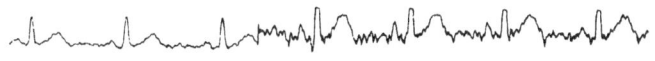

The transistor is a solid-state device which has the advantage that it is small, lightweight and does not consume much energy.

Usually a transistor consists of three layers of semiconductor material (see Chapter 4), normally silicon, each layer having its own specific built-in impurities by which its conduction is controlled.

A current through the three layers can be adjusted by a voltage between two of them. The layer where the current enters the device is called the 'emitter', the layer where the current leaves the device is called the 'collector', and the layer between the emitter and the collector is called the 'base' of the transistor. A voltage applied between the base and the emitter will adjust the current from emitter to collector. If this current flows through a resistor, then a voltage appears across that resistor. This voltage

Fig. 7.3. Various types of transistors and the symbol for a transistor.

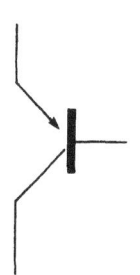

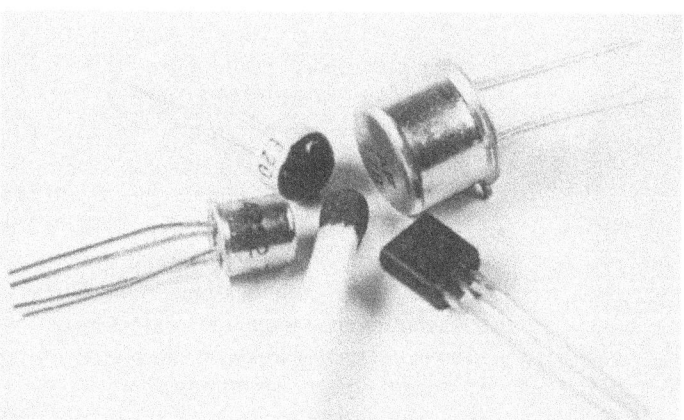

Fig. 7.4. A circuit diagram of a one-stage transistor amplifier; $V_{out}/V_{in} = A$.

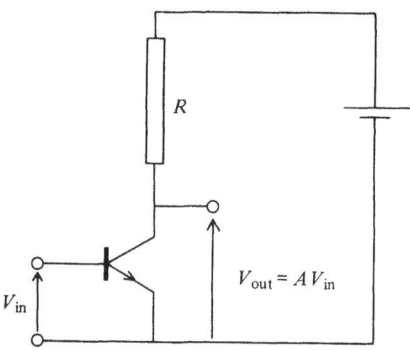

R

V_{in}

$V_{out} = A V_{in}$

will generally have a higher amplitude than the amplitude of the emitter-to-base voltage. Thus an input voltage is transformed into an output voltage with a higher amplitude, that is, the input voltage is multiplied by a certain gain factor, A.

If one transistor–resistor combination does not result in an adequate gain, then the output voltage can be amplified repeatedly. Amplifier stages can be connected in series, increasing the total gain to any required value.

The transistors and resistors necessary for an amplifier with a certain gain can be directly constructed in one piece of silicon, with the proper connections to each other already built in. This results in a complete amplifier with, for instance, a gain of 10 000. This is called an integrated circuit.

The technology of manufacturing integrated circuits is the most important development of recent years, especially with respect to electromedical instrumentation. Thanks to integrated circuit technology it is possible to make very small electronic amplifiers which can be built into the human body.

In addition to the decreased size, compared with the early valve amplifiers, it is also a great advantage that transistor amplifiers do not consume much energy and can be supplied by rather small voltages. This means that they can be battery operated, which is an advantage from the view of patient safety (see Chapter 12).

Amplifiers always have to be connected between a voltage

Fig. 7.5. Examples of integrated circuits.

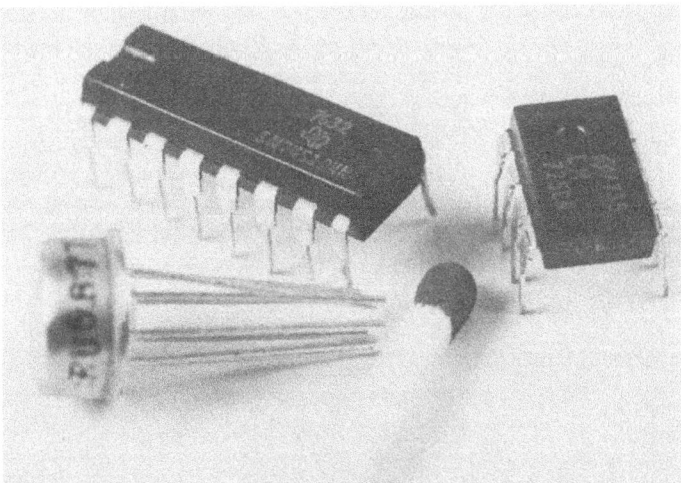

source and recorder or other display device. These connections are provided by cables and connectors and, because the amplifier itself has become smaller and smaller, the logical tendency is to use very thin cables and small connectors. As already mentioned in Chapter 5, miniaturisation demands extra attention from the user, because microcomponents are more fragile than the larger ones.

An actual amplifier is not normally recognisable as a separate device because it is built in to a particular piece of equipment, such as an electrocardiograph. The function of the amplifying section of any electromedical instrument is so important that it is very useful to consider this in more detail.

A problem with every amplifying system is that other voltages besides the voltage of interest, are often amplified and may seriously disturb the recording. This effect can be caused by capacitive coupling between the amplifier input leads and any conducting materials in the vicinity. If one of these materials, for instance a wire, has an alternating voltage with respect to the input lead of the amplifier, then this voltage will also be measured, because a capacitor behaves as a conductor for alternating currents. As every room usually contains several electric power lines from the mains supply, most measuring devices are affected by the capacitive coupling with the mains. This is the reason that recordings of electrophysiological signals are often disturbed by mains-frequency 'hum'.

One remedy for this interference is to use coaxial cables which are shielded by a flexible woven coating of conducting material connected to earth. The inner lead of the shielded cable is now capacitively coupled only with its own shield, which has a voltage of zero if it is properly connected to earth, resulting in no voltage pick-up by the input of the amplifier. If, however, the end of the shielded cable is connected to a patient by means of an electrode, then again a large capacitive coupling between the input of the amplifier and the mains supply is created, because the patient now acts as one 'plate' of a capacitor, the other 'plate' being formed by the electric power lines in the vicinity of the patient.

This can be remedied by shielding the whole patient by means of a cage of iron or copper gauze. This is often done for EEG

Fig. 7.6. A general registration set-up consisting of a transducer, an amplifier and a recorder.

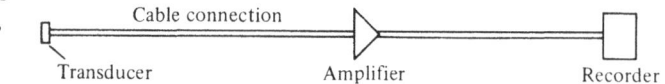

Fig. 7.7. A schematic diagram of mains inter-ference as a result of capacitive coupling between the mains and the input lead of an amplifier.

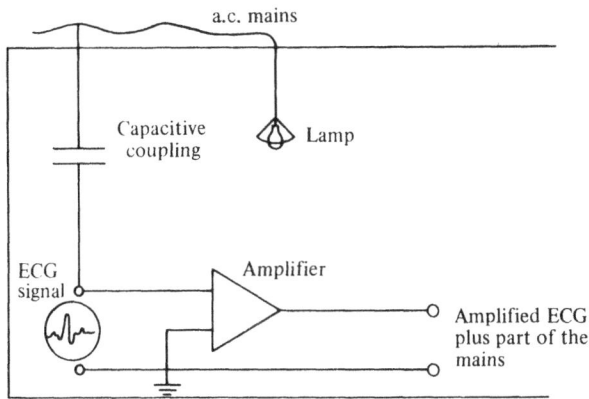

Fig. 7.8. (a) A schematic representation of a shielded cable. (b) As Fig. 7.7, but now with the capacitive coupling between the mains and the patient, a situation which always exists in spite of the use of shielded cables.

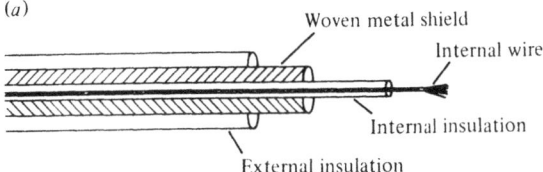

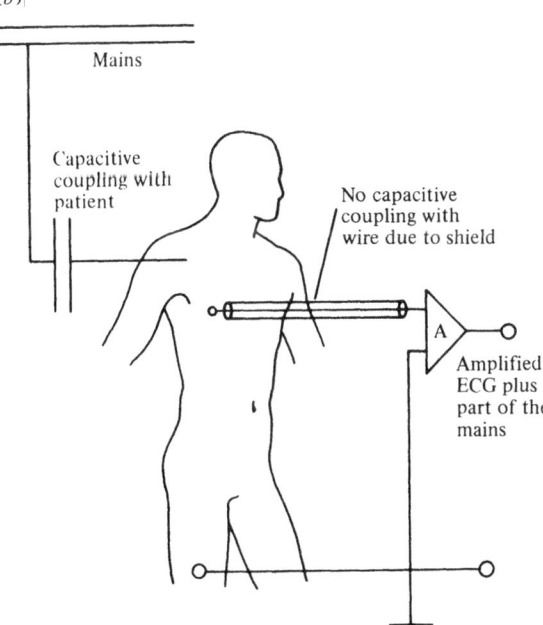

measurements, where a whole room may be screened for EEG analysis, producing a so-called 'Faraday cage'. In many cases the use of a cage is not practicable and for these cases a special type of amplifier has been developed, the differential amplifier.

The invention of the differential amplifier is based on the idea that the whole body can be considered as one capacitor 'plate' with good conducting properties, with the power lines in the vicinity as the other 'plate'. This means that the whole body also carries a voltage at mains frequency with respect to earth.

No difference exists in the amplitude of this voltage between two points of the body or, in other words, the body has a 'common-mode signal' due to its capacitive coupling with the mains. If an ECG voltage is generated between two points, this can thus be considered as a differential voltage between those points, which also have a common-mode voltage at mains frequency. The differential amplifier has been developed for this special combination of voltages, and has the property of amplifying only differential and not common-mode signals. Only in this way can ECGs be measured without mains hum.

Differential amplifiers are, in practice, not ideal in their rejection of common-mode signals. Their rejection is limited to a factor of 10 000 or 100 000 to 1 with respect to the amplitude of

Fig. 7.9. A diagram of the application of a differential amplifier.

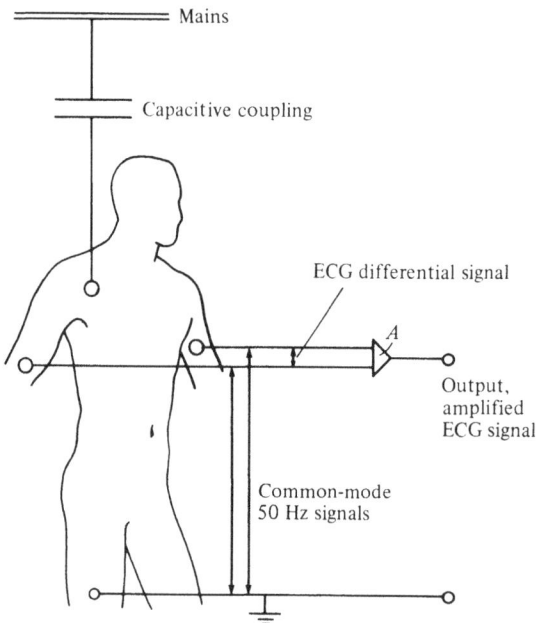

the differential voltage. This factor is called the common-mode rejection ratio, CMRR.

If, for example, the built-in amplifier of an electrocardiograph has a gain of 1000 for differential input voltages, while common-mode signals are at the same time attenuated by a factor of 100, then the CMRR is 100 000. Thus a common-mode signal of 1 V appears at the output of the amplifier with an amplitude of 10 mV. At the same time the ECG of 1 mV is amplified up to 1 V, which means that the level of common-mode signal is 1% of the ECG amplitude, a reasonable value.

If the common-mode signal was 10 V in the example mentioned above, then the hum signal would have been 10%, which is not permissible. It is thus of great advantage to make the common-mode voltage in the first place as small as possible. This can be done by a proper earthing of the patient. The next example will explain this with real values.

If it is assumed that a patient has a capacitance of about 100 pF with respect to the electric power lines in his vicinity, then he is in fact connected to the mains of 240 volts by means of an impedance of about 30 MΩ (100 pF is 30 MΩ for 50 Hz). If the patient's impedance to earth is also 30 MΩ, then his common-mode voltage will be ½ × 240 V = 120 V, which is of course much too high. If the impedance to earth is made as low as 1 kΩ, using a well-connected earth electrode, then the common-mode voltage is 1/30 000 × 240 V = 8 mV, which is of course much more acceptable. A differential amplifier with a CMRR of 10 000

Fig. 7.10. A schematic diagram of an earthed patient with resulting common-mode voltage as function of the impedance of the earth electrode.

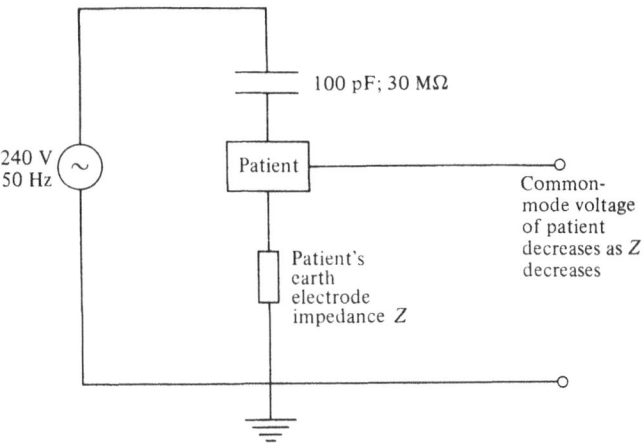

will now be sufficient to measure an ECG of 1 mV without any distortion. The manufacturer of ECG recorders uses this as a starting point for the development of the built-in amplifier, which means that the user is obliged to fulfil the conditions of proper earthing. The example obviously illustrates that a poor earth contact, i.e. a relatively high earth-electrode impedance, may result in a high level of distortion. This fault should not be ascribed to the equipment but to the user.

Of course, poor contact at one of the measuring electrodes will also have the same effect. An extreme example occurs when one of the electrodes is disconnected. Then both input connections of the differential amplifier do not receive the mains-frequency voltage as a common signal, but rather as a difference, which will be amplified, resulting in a large mains-frequency signal at the output.

Summarising, a differential amplifier always has three leads, two actual input leads and one earth lead, all of which have to be connected in order to make the maximum use of the differential configuration.

Under certain circumstances, even the application of a differential amplifier is not sufficient to suppress interference from signals outside the body completely, especially if the signals to be measured have very small amplitudes, as in the case of EEG measurements. Then the maximum obtainable CMRR is often

Fig. 7.11. The application of a differential amplifier will result in amplification of part of the mains if one electrode makes a poor contact (electrode no. 1).

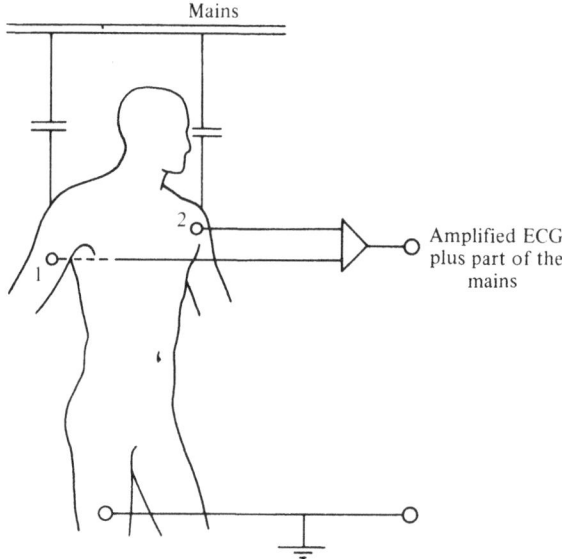

not sufficient. This is the reason that routine EEG recordings are sometimes made in a shielded room, a Faraday cage, and even then the electrodes have to be placed very carefully in order to prevent interference.

Interference does sometimes appear in recordings even if the best differential amplifier is used and very carefully applied. This is due to the presence of high-frequency equipment in the vicinity of the place of measurement. The equipment used for coagulation and diathermy transmits high-frequency signals over a long distance. The capacitive coupling between a patient and this apparatus has a relatively low impedance, since the impedance of a capacitor is inversely proportional to the frequency (see Chapter 5). This means that the common-mode voltage of the patient can be very high, and that high-frequency currents of a relatively high value will flow through the patient.

Since the patient does not have a resistance of zero ohm, this current through the patient will create a voltage across the body. This means that an unwanted signal is generated between the measuring electrodes, which is amplified by the same gain as the voltage to be measured. Although the interference signal has a high frequency, which can be filtered out, the problem is that low-frequency signals, especially mains frequency, are always carried by the high-frequency signal. These parts of the transmitted signal result in the observed distortion.

Even the best differential amplifier cannot solve this problem. If differential signals have to be measured between two points, then of course all differential signals which are present are ampli-

Fig. 7.12. Voltages generated across the body due to diathermy equipment will be amplified in the same way as the original bioelectric voltage (ECG).

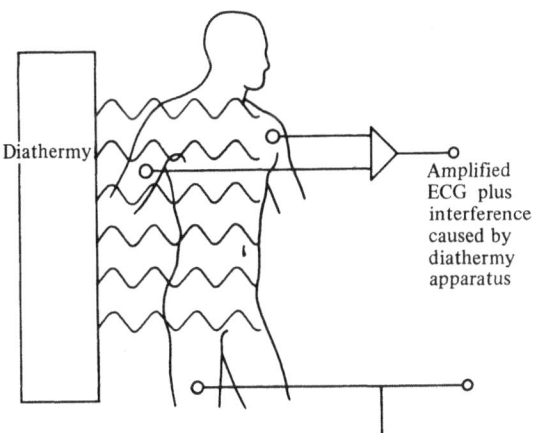

fied. The only remedy in this case is to remove the high-frequency equipment from the vicinity of the patient or vice versa.

Note that owing to the long transmission distance of high-frequency signals, interference can occur from high-frequency equipment in use in another room, next to, above or below the room in which the measurements are being made. This must always be taken into account if a problem with persistent mains-frequency interference is encountered.

After these special features of amplifiers, two more general phenomena should be described in relation to the application of amplifiers.

Even if the input leads of an amplifier are connected together, so that there is no input voltage, the output may still show a small signal, which is generated by the internal components of the amplifier itself. The resulting signal usually cannot be characterised by a mean amplitude or frequency, and is called 'noise'. The manufacturer of an amplifier has usually developed it for a special function and may guarantee that, for that particular task, the amplifier noise is sufficiently low. Using the amplifier for other applications for which it was not designed may result in serious noise problems.

Besides noise, an amplifier always generates a direct voltage at its output. This may drift away from zero volt, at which value the amplifier has usually been adjusted. This drift, often due to the changing temperature of the equipment, appears as a shift in the baseline of the recording. An amplifier is therefore usually provided with a control for the adjustment of the d.c. level at its output, mostly indicated with terms like 'baseline correction', 'balance', 'zero', or 'position'.

As the level of the output of an amplifier is a function of temperature, so the gain of an amplifier may sometimes also be influenced by temperature. This is the reason that amplifiers usually have a control for gain adjustment, which may only be used for calibration of the amplifier. This control is therefore usually only adjustable by means of a screwdriver. It is generally designated 'CAL'.

8. Recording systems

In practice, a measured signal nearly always consists of a voltage which has to be displayed in order that it may be interpreted for diagnosis. Sometimes the signal is made audible, by means of an amplifier and a loudspeaker, but mostly it is presented in a visible form. In principle this can be done in two ways: by means of an analogue representation or a digital representation of the amplitude of the signal. With an analogue indication the voltage is usually represented by the needle of a meter, which moves along a calibrated scale.

In fact, all these meters are voltmeters and can be likened to an electric motor with limited rotational properties. The rotation of a coil in a magnetic field is balanced by means of a spring. Using a suitable internal series resistor, the maximum deflection of the needle, which is connected to the moving coil, can be adapted to the voltage range to be measured. The accuracy of this type of meter is not very good, especially if the meter setting has to be observed from relatively long distances, for instance from the end of a bed.

It is easier to read displayed data from a long distance when digital techniques are used. Here the amplitude of a signal is directly given in digits by means of illuminated figures, as in a pocket calculator.

Fig. 8.1. An example of an analogue meter, in this case a current meter calibrated in mA.

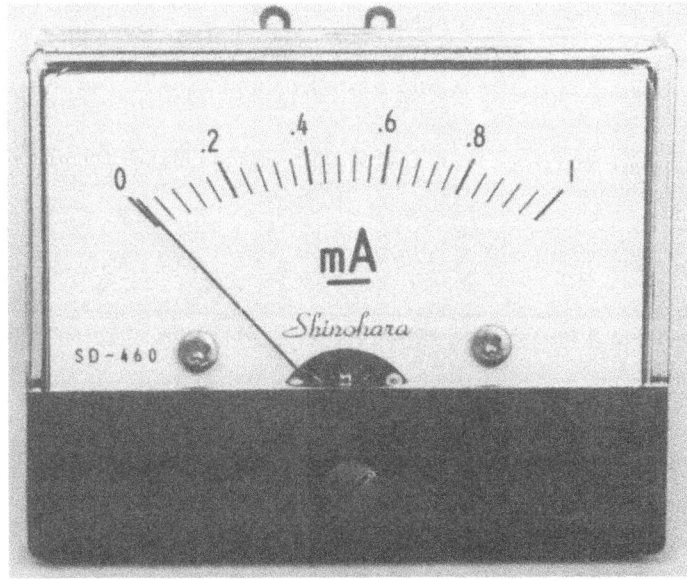

It will be obvious that the accuracy is now increased, because a digital meter can also show digits after the decimal point. It is possible for instance to display a pH of 7.732, which is not possible with most analogue meters, where pH = 7.7 is in this case the maximum possible accuracy that could be observed.

Both types of meters are generally provided with built-in amplifiers, but much more electronic circuitry is necessary for the digital meter because of its conversion and processing of data.

Both types of instrument can only be used for displaying static or quasi-static signals (with slow variations). Only mean values can be displayed, while varying values can only be followed if they are of very low frequency. These meters, therefore, cannot be used for dynamic studies, as for instance for investigation of the ECG complex. Also the voltmeters described above do not store signals, which means that only instantaneous values can be read from them without any record of the previous values. In other words trends cannot be measured with normal analogue and digital meters.

Oscilloscopes and graphic recorders are used for measuring dynamic signals, as well as providing storage facilities. An oscilloscope consists of a cathode-ray tube the screen of which can be seen by the user, as with an ordinary TV screen. As well as this cathode-ray tube, an oscilloscope has three more essential units, the input amplifier, the time-base unit and a built-in power supply.

Fig. 8.2. An example of a digital meter, in this case an a.c. or d.c. volt- or current-meter and an ohm-meter.

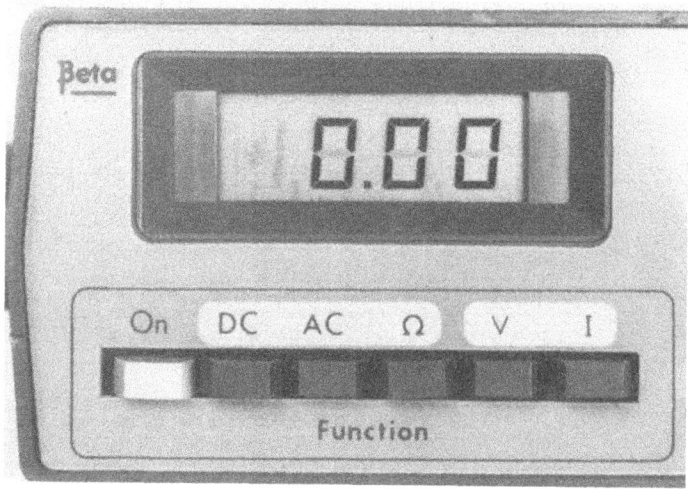

In the cathode-ray tube an 'electron gun' projects a thin stream of electrons on to the fluorescent screen, which lights up at the place where the electrons strike it. This can be seen as a small spot of light whose intensity can be controlled by applying a voltage to an internal grid in the tube. This voltage is usually controlled by a potentiometer which can be externally adjusted. The designation for this control is normally 'intensity'. The size and fineness of the spot can be adjusted with a 'focus' control.

The usefulness of the oscilloscope is derived from the fact that the light spot at the screen can be made to move along the screen in a horizontal as well as a vertical direction. To do this, two pairs of plates are mounted inside the cathode-ray tube, perpendicular to each other inside the tube. A voltage applied to these plates deflects the beam of electrons by means of the effect described in Chapter 2, that is, electrons are attracted to a positive and repelled by a negative plate.

The plates which control the horizontal deflection are connected to a voltage which has a saw-tooth character, with a set period. The result is that the light spot moves from left to right in a certain time, fixed by the period of the saw-tooth voltage. This

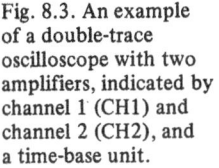

Fig. 8.3. An example of a double-trace oscilloscope with two amplifiers, indicated by channel 1 (CH1) and channel 2 (CH2), and a time-base unit.

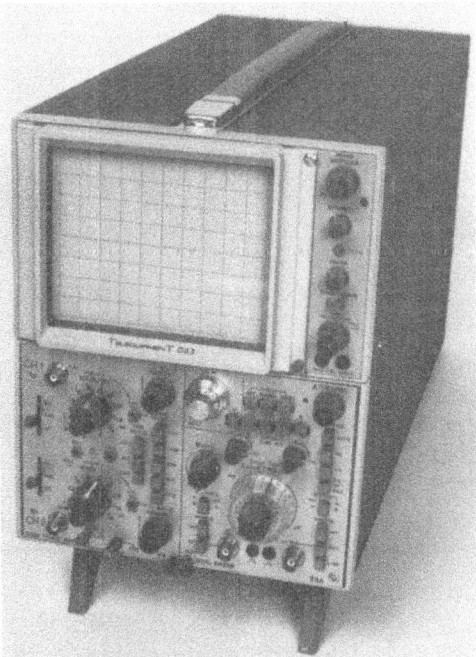

gives the impression of a moving spot if the writing speed is low, or a horizontal line on the screen if the writing speed is high. The writing-speed control unit is often called the 'time-base'. The text at the control for adjusting the writing speed is therefore a time division, for instance 100 ms/div., which makes it possible to interpret the horizontal axis of the oscilloscope screen directly as a time axis. The saw-tooth (time-base) voltage is generated by a 'sweep generator' in the oscilloscope.

The plates that control the vertical deflection are connected to the output of the amplifier that amplifies the signal to be investigated, for instance an ECG voltage. This means that during the movement of the light-spot in the horizontal direction, a deflection occurs in the vertical direction as a function of the amplitude of the ECG signal. The amplitude on the screen can be controlled by the gain control of the amplifier. By adding a direct voltage to the output of the signal amplifier, a constant deflection in the vertical direction can be achieved, thus making it possible to control the position of the trace on the screen. A control marked 'vertical deflection' determines the position of the base-line on the screen.

In order to ensure that a periodic signal always appears on the screen at the same place during each sweep of the time-base, thus preventing the signal wandering along the screen, the sweep always has to start at a moment which has a fixed relationship to the time intervals of the signal to be displayed. Thus a certain synchronisation is necessary, which is also called a triggering of the time-base. Usually this triggering occurs internally in the oscilloscope, but sometimes it may also be activated by an externally applied signal which then fixes the moment of triggering the time-base.

Fig. 8.4. A schematic representation of a cathode-ray tube.

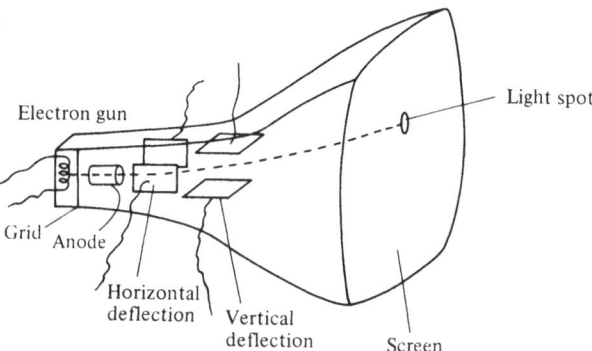

When recording the ECG, for example, the horizontal deflection is usually a slow one so that several complexes may be viewed at once. In this case synchronisation of the sweep is not necessary.

The fluorescent properties of the screen are obtained from a chemical coating on the inner side of the tube. There are different chemical coatings available, but a coating which has a long persistence is often selected for use in medical equipment. This means that the moving spot of light leaves a trace that remains visible for some time. This means that a signal can be compared with one or two previous signals, as is often necessary with an ECG recording. Each ECG complex can now be related to the previous complexes so that rhythm changes can be studied.

Some oscilloscopes also have a variable persistence, which can be controlled manually. The persistence can last so long that the signal during one sweep can be stored on the screen and so can be studied for as long as necessary. This type of oscilloscope is called a 'storage oscilloscope' but no electronic memory is contained within the instrument. If the recording has to be stored for later comparison with other recordings, it must be photographed, and for this purpose special cameras are available, which can be attached to the oscilloscope. More special features of the application of an oscilloscope for monitoring will be described in Chapter 10.

Graphic recorders are also frequently used for recording of biomedical signals. The signals are recorded by a pen on a moving strip of paper so, in general, two basic parts can be distinguished in a paper recorder, namely the writing section and the paper transportation.

The paper is transported by means of an electric motor driving a gearbox, and often a number of paper speeds can be selected. As the paper is divided by lines into sections of, for instance, millimetres or centimetres, and the speed of the paper is known in millimetres or centimetres per second, the length of a written signal can be expressed directly in units of time. The paper-speed control is thus essentially the same as the time-base control of an oscilloscope.

A variety of possibilities are available for the writing system, each with its own advantages and disadvantages. With an ink writer, a pen is used through which ink is drawn from an ink reservoir. The pen itself is connected to a deflection motor, which is essentially a rigid analogue voltmeter. A moving coil in a magnetic field is balanced with a spring and the resulting deflection is pro-

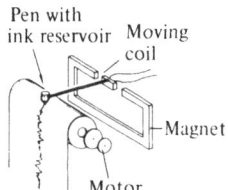

Fig. 8.5. A schematic representation of a pen recorder.

portional to an applied voltage. As the whole moving part is rather bulky and also the necessary contact between the pen and the paper is rather heavy, an ink writer cannot record very rapid signals. This means that ink writers can only be used for recording low-frequency signals with a maximum of about 70 Hz. For signals within this range, for instance EEG signals, the ink writer can be used to good advantage. If the recording system is only occasionally used, the drying-out of the pens may be inconvenient. Using felt-tip writers may partly solve this problem, although they dry out too.

An ink writer which works by spraying ink on to the paper is suitable for recording higher frequencies, up to about 700 Hz. The jet-pen, which is again connected to a kind of pen motor, is very lightly constructed and because it does not make contact with the paper, its movements can be much faster. Again the system has to be used regularly to prevent problems with drying of ink in the system.

For still higher frequencies, for instance those found in intramuscular EMG registrations, recorders have been developed in which the weight of the moving parts has been reduced even more. In such recorders, a small mirror is mounted on a moving coil meter and a beam of light is deflected through an angle proportional to the voltage applied to the coil. The deflected light beam is recorded on film. For convenience of operation under daylight conditions, ultraviolet light and ultraviolet-sensitive paper is used. This paper is automatically developed within a few minutes in daylight. The recordings have to be stored in the dark because they will be affected by sunlight or other ultraviolet light sources, causing them to fade gradually. Fixation with a special spray may help prevent this.

A writing system has been developed which does not give rise to problems with ink or light. This system is the thermowriter. Special paper has to be used for this system. The paper has a white layer of wax on top of a black under-surface. This wax can be melted easily by a stylus heated by an electric current which flows through a resistive element at the tip of the stylus arm and which makes contact with the waxed paper. This system requires little maintenance, and is generally used in electrocardiographs. The frequency band is again limited because of the contact friction between the stylus and the paper, although this system will work up to 100 Hz. Contact pressure can be adjusted to make it optimal for any stylus temperature. As the frequency band required influences the choice of stylus pressure and stylus heat, the recorder has to be checked frequently to ensure that these are correct.

Note that, in general, the complete system of amplifier and recorder has a frequency band within the limits of the separate component parts. A system with an amplifier which is suitable for 10–100 Hz and a recorder for 0–100 Hz, but with a wrong adjustment so that the frequency band is limited to 40 Hz, will only record signals from 10–40 Hz. Therefore a recording system always has to be calibrated as a whole.

Another method of storing electrical signals is on magnetic tape, either reel to reel or, more often nowadays, a cassette recorder. The data can be reproduced at any time as electrical signals by playing back the tape. This is a great advantage in comparison with paper tape recorders, where the signals cannot be reproduced as electrical signals for later processing.

Magnetic tape recorders in use for music and speech do not have a frequency band suitable for many biomedical signals. Special tape recorders have been developed, with an adequate frequency band and often with many channels for simultaneous recordings.

Besides voltages generated directly from the human body or indirectly by means of transducers, processed voltages can also be recorded. If, for example, only the heart rate is of interest, then the amplified ECG signal may be applied directly to an electronic counter and only the output of this device recorded, in order to be able to obtain an indication of the trend in the heart rate.

Such processing may only involve simple filtering, but even so the original signal can never be reproduced from the recording.

Fig. 8.6. With a series connection of an amplifier and a recorder, the frequency band is determined by the combination of both instruments.

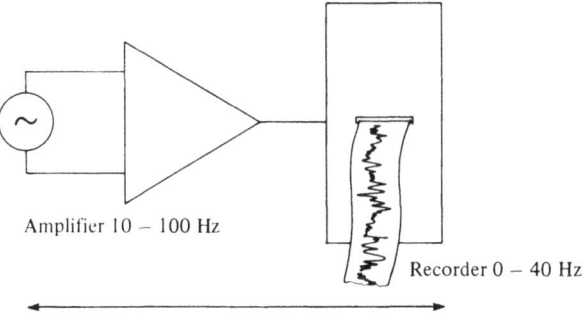

Amplifier 10 – 100 Hz

Recorder 0 – 40 Hz

Frequency band 10–40 Hz

Before recording any signal, one has to consider what information will be of interest later on. If, for instance, a frequency analysis has to be carried out on data recorded on magnetic tape, the actual recording must be made on a tape recorder capable of detecting and storing all the necessary frequencies.

Fig. 8.7. A schematic diagram of a heart-rate monitor.

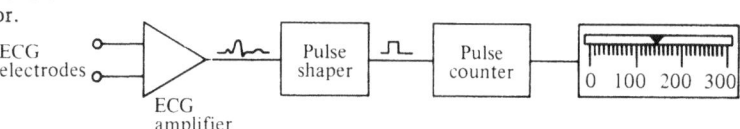

ECG electrodes

ECG amplifier

Pulse shaper

Pulse counter

0   100 200 300

9. Electromedical measuring systems for ECG, EEG and EMG

In previous chapters, reference has been made to the measurement of biopotentials without referring to those characteristics of the measuring instruments which can lead to error in certain circumstances.

Each measuring instrument, whether it is an analogue voltmeter, a digital voltmeter or the amplifier of a recorder, has a certain internal resistance which appears across the input leads. This resistance is called the input resistance of the device; if alternating voltages are considered it is better to describe it as the input impedance. If the voltage of a source has to be measured it should be realised that the measuring instrument has a certain internal impedance. When measuring biological potentials the source impedance is usually fixed by the impedance of the electrodes which connect the voltage source to the measuring device. As already mentioned in Chapter 5, two impedances connected in series will behave as a voltage divider. This means that only part of the voltage to be measured appears across the input impedance of the instrument, resulting in a smaller value being measured than was expected. This may lead to serious discrepancies in the recording. If, for example, the input impedance of an ECG amplifier is equal to the sum of the electrode impedances of the applied electrodes, only half of the ECG amplitude will be measured.

In general, a measurement accuracy of 1% is sufficient, which means that the input impedance of the measuring device has to be at least 100 times larger than the maximum expected value of the combined electrode impedances. Since electrode impedances of the order of a few thousand ohms can be achieved by careful electrode placement (see Chapter 6), about 5 kΩ for a pair of electrodes, measuring devices with an input impedance of 500 kΩ give a satisfactory accuracy. In order to guarantee the required accuracy of 1% the user of the apparatus has to comply with the

Fig. 9.1. A diagram of an amplifier with input impedance Z_{input} to which electrodes are connected with impedances Z_{e1} and Z_{e2}.

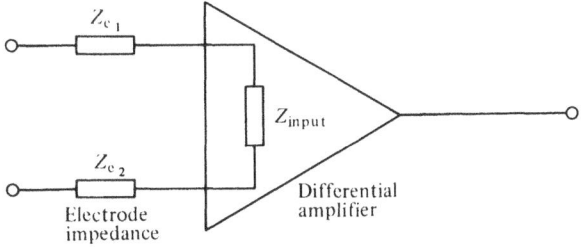

operating conditions by ensuring that the impedance for each electrode is 2.5 kΩ or smaller. Here again understanding and careful use of the equipment is the main factor for successful measurements.

Another problem may result from the parallel impedance between the input leads of the amplifier. If the input impedance of a measuring device is guaranteed by the manufacturer to be 500 kΩ, but in practice this impedance is shunted by 100 kΩ, then the resulting impedance is smaller than 100 kΩ. This again makes the voltage division unfavourable, decreasing the amplitude of the measured voltage. Such a shunt impedance may be caused by careless use of electrode paste which may form a conducting path across the skin between the measuring electrodes. Sweat may also form such a shunt, as often occurs during exercise tests.

In addition to these possible external sources of error, other faults may also occur due to internal sources of interference. As already mentioned, the electrode–tissue contact behaves as a voltage source in series with the biopotential to be measured. Thus electrode potentials will be measured and amplified with the same gain as the biopotential of interest. Electrode potentials may show drift due to polarisation of the electrodes, but may also change rapidly due to movement of the electrodes themselves. The only way to get rid of these unwanted potentials is by using a high-pass filter. Unfortunately, as already mentioned, some lower-frequency components of the signal of interest are then also filtered out, so the use of such filtering can be allowed only if low-frequency distortion of the signal is permissible. This is often the case with intensive-care equipment where an ECG measurement is usually done only to provide information about the patient's heart rate. Time constants of 0.3 s are generally in use in this case (low cut-off frequency of about 0.6 Hz). The

Fig. 9.2. As Fig. 9.1, but with an additional shunt impedance Z_{shunt}, due to sweat or spoiled electrode jelly, lowering the amplifier input impedance, Z_{input}.

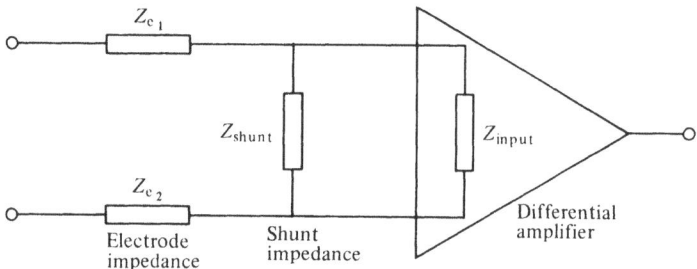

control by which this type of filter can be introduced is usually designated 'monitor'. For an accurate ECG diagnosis the filter has to be switched out, resulting in a time constant of 3.2 s.

Another source of trouble occurs if more than one bio-electric voltage source is part of the measuring circuit. In principle this is always the case, but problems occur when these sources are simultaneously active. The result is a mixture of the contributions of several sources, which can only be separated by filtering. Again this filtering gives rise to the problem that essential frequency components of the required signal may be filtered out. In the first instance, it is recommended to arrange the measurement conditions so that only one voltage source is active during the time of measuring.

EMG activity in an ECG recording must first be countered by trying to keep the patient relaxed if he is tensed, or by keeping him warm if he is shivering. Only if the EMG activity is excessive should a filter be used; when it is this should always be noted on the recording.

ECG

After these general remarks about the measurement of bio-electric potentials we will concentrate on ECG recording, which is essentially the recording of the electrical activity of the heart by means of body-surface electrodes. The recorder developed for this purpose – the electrocardiograph – will also be considered.

At any instant during the activation of the heart the total activity of the individual cells may be represented by a resultant electrical vector. As activation proceeds, this vector changes in

Fig. 9.3. Example of ECG registration with 'monitor' off (lower trace) and 'monitor' on (upper trace). The upper trace clearly shows less influence of EMG activity and electrode movement artifact, but also a decreased value of the R-wave.

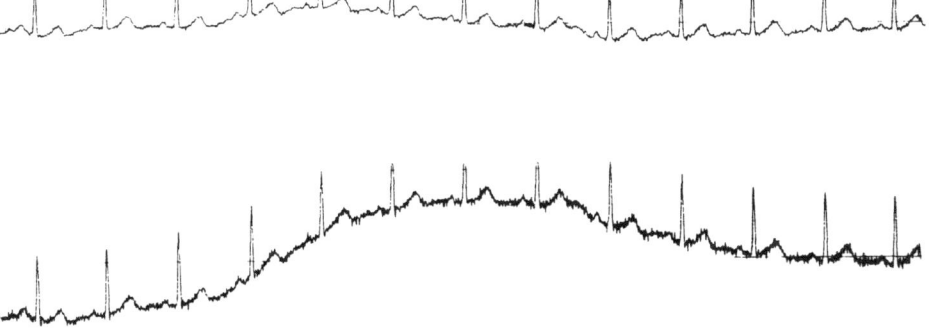

both magnitude and direction. In principle an infinite number of places on the surface of the body may be chosen to record this activity, resulting in any number of ECG configurations. In order to be able to compare different ECGs, cardiologists have agreed on a limited number of measuring sites and conventions.

Since the depolarisation vector moves in three dimensions, it is customary to record its projection on to each of three mutually perpendicular planes in turn. These are termed the frontal, transverse and sagittal planes.

In the frontal plane, six leads are normally recorded, from electrodes connected to the arms and the left leg. Differential amplifiers are used with the reference attached to an electrode on the right leg, which may or may not be earthed.

Three of the leads are termed 'bipolar', as they record the activity between two electrodes attached to the patient. The convention obeyed is as follows:

> Lead I   recorded between left arm and right arm;
> Lead II recorded between left leg and right arm;
> Lead III recorded between left leg and left arm.

The remaining three leads in the frontal plane are termed 'unipolar', as they record the activity between one electrode on the patient and a reference point formed by summing the potentials on the arms and the left leg. When the electrode whose activity is being recorded is disconnected from this reference point this has the effect of increasing the amplitude of the signal. This results in the 'augmented' unipolar leads in the frontal plane. Thus:

> aVR: measurement between right arm and left arm—left leg connection.

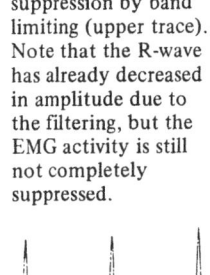

Fig. 9.4. Example of ECG registration disturbed by EMG (lower trace) with EMG suppression by band limiting (upper trace). Note that the R-wave has already decreased in amplitude due to the filtering, but the EMG activity is still not completely suppressed.

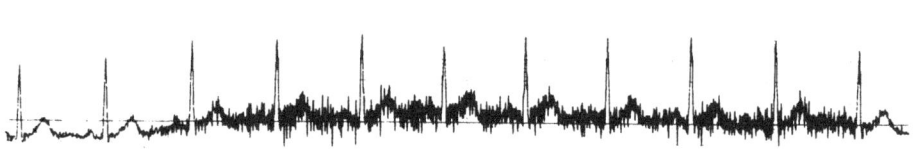

Fig. 9.5. A diagram of bipolar and unipolar limb leads, with corresponding registrations.

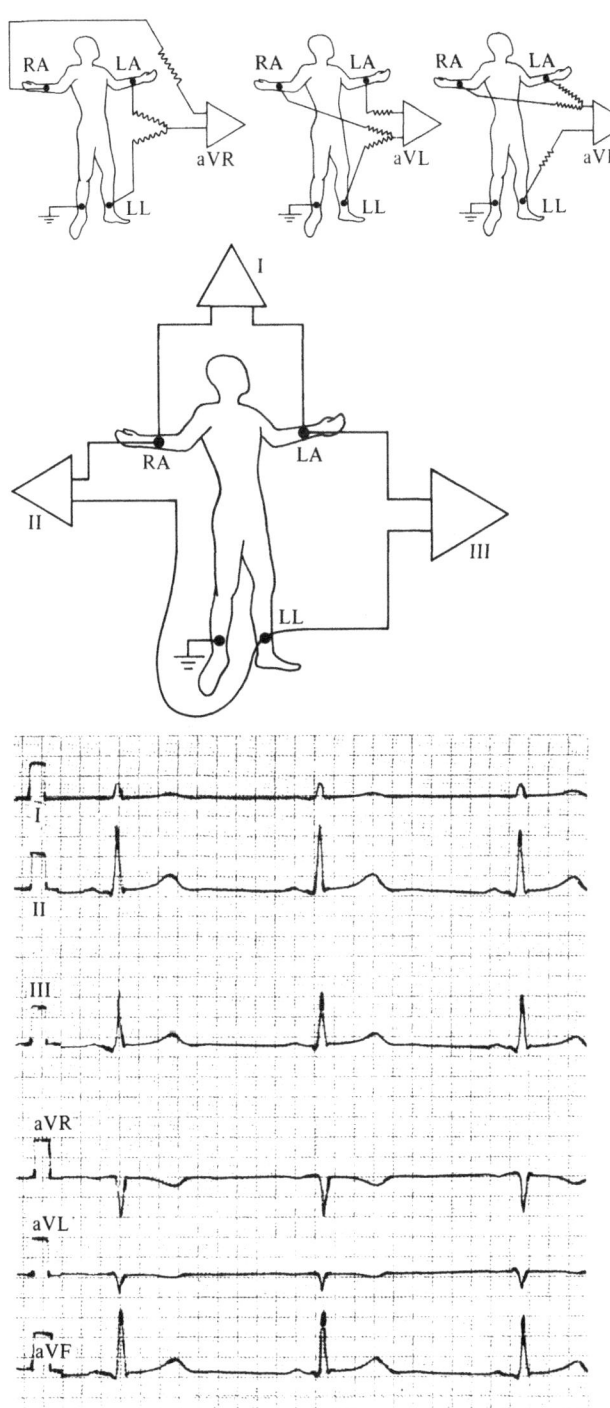

aVL: measurement between left arm and left leg—right arm connection.

aVF: measurement between left leg and left arm—right arm connection.

In order to record the projections on to the horizontal plane, six standard electrode positions are used, termed V1 to V6, in which case the electrodes are positioned as follows:

V1: fourth intercostal space, at right sternal margin.

V2: fourth intercostal space, at left sternal margin.

V3: midway between V2 and V4.

V4: fifth intercostal space, at midclavicular line.

V5: same level as V4, on anterior axillary line.

V6: same level as V4, on midaxillary line.

During the recording of these 'precordial' leads, the amplifier is connected between each electrode in turn and a reference point formed by the connection of the right and left arm and the left leg.

Recording the projections of the cardiac vector on to the sagittal plane is not normally done in routine electrocardiography, as this involves the use of an intra-oesophageal electrode.

During these measurements, when the lead selector switch is turned to each position, the relevant electrodes are automatically connected together in the correct combinations.

In order to prevent mistakes in connecting the electrodes with the appropriate input lead of the electrocardiograph, a colour code has been introduced for the different leads, as shown in Table 9.1.

It is conventional to use a total of twelve standard leads from a patient. From these combinations a skilled cardiologist can detect the condition of the heart using his experience and physiological knowledge about correlations between symptomatic complaints and ECG patterns. It is absolutely essential therefore that dis-

Table 9.1. *Colour coding of ECG electrode leads*

Connection	Colour	Indication
Right arm	White	RA
Left arm	Black	LA
Left leg	Red	LL
Right leg	Green	RL
Chest	Brown	C

Fig. 9.6. Unipolar chest
leads with corresponding
registrations.

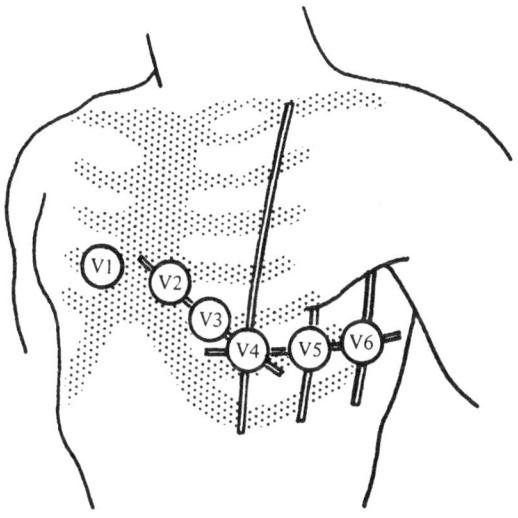

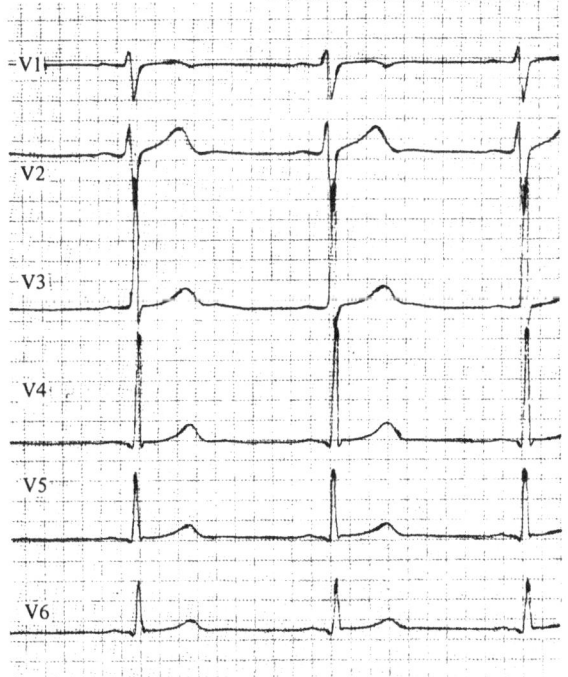

tortion caused by the operation of the cardiograph should not occur, for instance from filtering. Also the cardiologist has to know which lead was registered. Often the position of the lead selector switch is printed on the paper strip by a marker which can be activated by a push-button, or is activated automatically as soon as a certain recording is started. Without this facility the particular lead must always be noted by the operator on the corresponding part of the recording paper.

Besides agreements concerning the locations of the electrodes and the twelve standard combinations of leads, agreements have also been reached about the speed of the paper. The most common speeds are 25 mm/s and 50 mm/s, resulting in time scales of respectively 1 mm = 40 ms and 1 mm = 20 ms.

In order to compare the amplitudes of recorded ECGs with each other, the voltage scale is also standardised so that 1 cm on the recording paper corresponds to 1 mV. For this reason every cardiograph has a push-button which generates a pulse of 1 mV between the input leads of the internal amplifier, by which the sensitivity can be calibrated. As already mentioned in Chapter 2, this pulse can also be used for verifying the required frequency bandwidth.

Summarising the description of an electrocardiograph given above and the general amplifier and recorder parameters as described in other chapters, the next typical operating controls are usually: on–off switch, lead-selector switch, stylus-position control, calibration marker, paper-speed control, stylus heat and sensitivity. In spite of this rather large number of controls, the electrocardiograph has become a diagnostic instrument almost as basic as the stethoscope or the blood-pressure cuff. It fully demonstrates that technical equipment can be helpful in medical care.

After this general description of the electrocardiograph, some more details about the essence of measuring a voltage between two points on the skin can be dealt with.

The measured voltage is always the result of a current flowing through the underlying tissue. The electrical current due to the electrical activity of the heart muscle is of course largest in the vicinity of the heart. This means that ECG activity cannot be measured between two points on the same arm because the electrical action of the heart does not result in current flowing lengthwise through the arm tissue. So when measuring between the arms it is immaterial at what place on the arm the electrode is located.

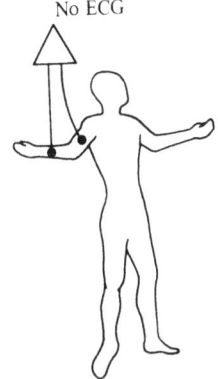

No ECG

Fig. 9.7. An ECG cannot be recorded between two places on the same limb.

The whole arm can be considered as an extension of the electrode lead to the actual place of measuring, which in this case is the shoulder.

As mentioned in Chapter 2, every voltage source has a polarity. This includes the ECG originating from the current flow between the shoulders. Therefore, exchanging the electrode connections between the arms will result in an ECG recording in which the usual waveform is inverted.

In reality the current flow around the heart varies not only in amplitude but also in direction, owing to the form and position of the heart in the chest. Such a current flow, whose amplitude and direction in space both vary, is termed a 'vector'. The projections of this vector on to three planes perpendicular to each other can be measured using the standard leads. If these three registrations are combined by means of a resistor network, then a curve can be drawn for each projection on the screen of an oscilloscope; this picture is called a vectorcardiogram (VCG).

Fig. 9.8. In principle, the ECG does not depend on the electrode position on the limbs.

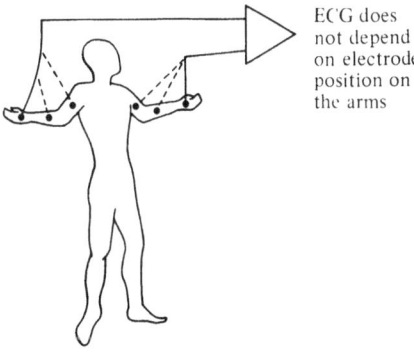

ECG does not depend on electrode position on the arms

Fig. 9.9. Exchanging electrode connections changes the polarity of the measured ECG.

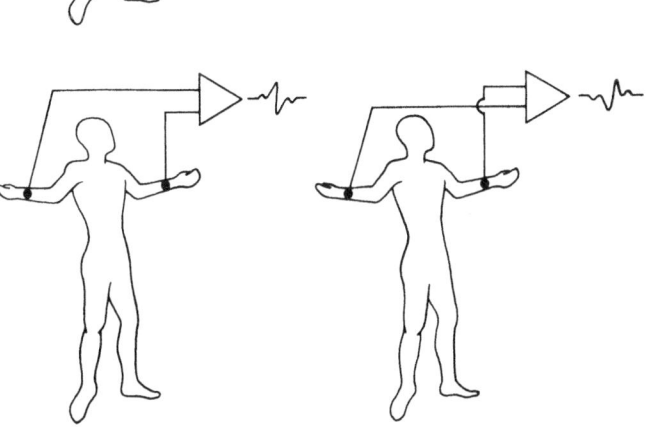

Vectorcardiographic equipment is more sophisticated than a normal electrocardiograph but its use can often help the cardiologist
to detect certain conditions which would not be obvious on a
standard electrocardiogram.

The electrocardiogram of a foetus can also be measured using a
lead on the maternal abdomen. This recording is called a foetal
electrocardiogram (FECG). The measuring problem mentioned in
the first section of this chapter is now intensified because besides
the voltage source of the foetal heart the voltage source of the
maternal heart (MECG) is also now included in the measuring
circuit.

In an FECG recording the maternal ECG is constantly present,
with a much higher amplitude. Sometimes special computer processing is used to overcome this problem, or else scalp electrodes
can be used on the foetal scalp, but this can only be done during
delivery.

EEG
The methods used to measure the electrical activity of organs
other than the heart are, in principle, just the same as in electrocardiography. Measuring the electrical activity of the brain
(electroencephalography, EEG) is also done by using electrodes at
standard locations, in this case on the scalp. The recorded rhythmic
waves are due to synchronised activity of neuronal cell groups.
Although their origin is not fully understood, experience of a
neurologist using the correlation between recorded EEG patterns
and neurological symptoms can lead to a useful diagnosis. In this
case too it has been agreed to use standard electrode locations.

The system most commonly in use is a standard harness of

Fig. 9.10. Example
of FECG registration
with an abdominal
lead with MECG as a
distortion.

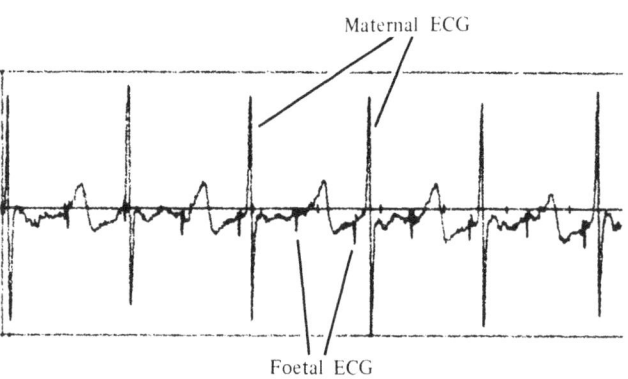

Maternal ECG

Foetal ECG

rubber straps by which twenty electrodes can be held in fixed positions, which are designated by letter and figure combinations. The letters are abbreviations of the names of lobes of the cerebellum: frontal = F, temporal = T, central = C, parietal = P and occipital = O.

Because the measured potentials are of the order of microvolts and in a frequency range from 0.1 Hz to about 100 Hz, special attention has to be paid to the construction and connection of the electrodes. Silver–silver chloride electrodes are used, and they have to be handled very carefully in order to prevent damage to the thin layer of silver chloride. They are, after careful preparation of the skin, attached with a quick-drying adhesive, usually collodion.

In order to prevent mains interference, routine EEG recordings may be performed in a shielded room (Faraday cage) free of electric equipment except any necessary pre-amplifiers, which are usually supplied with direct current. Even with the best differential amplifiers, strict requirements have to be fulfilled with respect to the equality of electrode impedances. Usually one can test the electrode impedances by means of a test generator built into the EEG equipment. Electrode impedances of the order of 1 kΩ are normal.

Some of the EEG equipment is provided with a facility for virtually earthing the patient. In this system the inverse of each common voltage is fed back to the patient, resulting in a consider-

Fig. 9.11. Standard electrode positions for EEG.

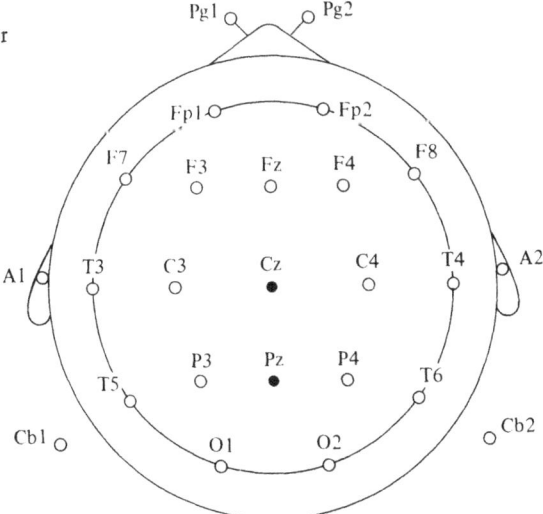

able decrease in the effective common voltage.

The EEG recorder itself is often a multichannel recorder, having up to 16 channels of a direct ink-writing type, or with an ink-jet writer. A large variety of combinations can be made using the twenty electrodes, and the results recorded by one of the channels. A large number of lead-selector switches can be found on the desk of an electroencephalograph recorder enabling the operator to choose from many combinations. The most common combinations are the unipolar mode, the average electrode mode and the bipolar mode. Often some standard modes are pro-grammed internally, so that one can switch from one mode to another simply by using one control of the EEG.

Besides the amplitude, the frequency of the recorded signal is also of interest. It is often useful to limit the band-width of a recording to the frequency band of the signal to be expected, for instance α-waves or δ-waves. In order to do this, a large number of filters can be switched in and out at the desk of an EEG recorder in order to focus on special rhythms. This can also be done automatically by means of a frequency analyser. Using this equipment the neurologist is provided directly with a recording of the frequency spectrum of the EEG.

A small computer is often used in an EEG department to help with this procedure. This set-up can be very helpful with routine EEG analysis but it appears that real pattern recognition is still the work of the neurologist.

The EEG recording again illustrates how electronic equipment can be used to provide diagnostic information not otherwise avail-able.

Besides the recording of spontaneous activity of the human brain, EEG patterns can also be evoked at certain places on the scalp by means of stimulating the corresponding senses. These recordings are called evoked responses and inform the neurologist about a whole functional system, for instance the visual faculty; this is stimulated by flashing light into the eyes. Small computers are often used for these measurements, to calculate the average response after several cycles of stimulation.

EMG

As well as measurement by ECG and EEG, skeletal muscle activity is often measured; this is known as electromyography (EMG). In principle the measurement of an EMG is the same as the other measurements, except that no standard leads are in use, owing to the large variety of muscles and the spread in anatomic performance. An EMG can be measured with surface electrodes in a differential mode, but also with needle electrodes which are inserted into the muscle. In the latter case the activities of single muscle fibres, called action potentials, can be measured, while with surface electrodes the summed activity of a large number of muscle fibres is recorded.

EMG potentials are of the order of millivolts and the frequency band for clinical use is from 10 Hz to 3 kHz, but up to 20 kHz may be recorded for research purposes. From the recordings, which are usually displayed on the screen of an oscilloscope,

Fig. 9.12. (a) Block diagram of EEG frequency analyser. (b) Typical example of EEG frequency analyser output for two separate cases: one recorded with a subject's eyes open and one with a subject's eyes closed, but with the subject awake.

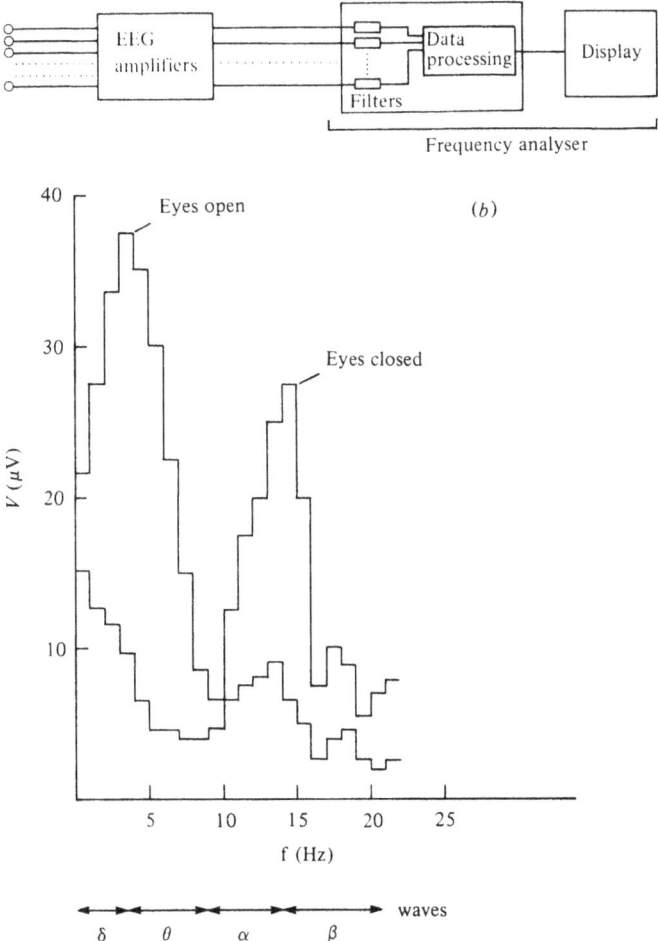

degeneration or other deviations of muscle function can be diagnosed.

The EMG activity measured at the muscles responsible for eye movement is called an electro-oculogram (EOG), while EMG activities associated with the peristaltic movements of the gastro-intestinal tract are called an electrogastrogram (EGG).

Bio-electric potentials generated in the retina of the eye by light stimulation can also be measured. The result is called an electroretinogram (ERG).

Fig. 9.13. Typical example of evoked-response experiment. (a) EEG recorded with scalp electrodes during repeated light flashes. (b) Part of the above waveform after analysis by a signal-averaging instrument, triggered by the light flash for 256 sweeps.

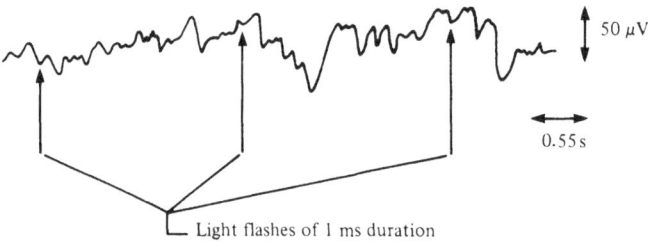

Light flashes of 1 ms duration

50 μV

0.55 s

(a)

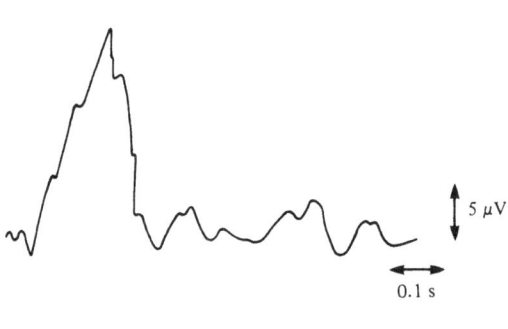

5 μV

0.1 s

(b)

Fig. 9.14. EMG recording with needle electrode (upper trace) and surface electrodes (lower trace). As can be seen, separate action potentials can be distinguished by using a needle electrode, while the measurement with surface electrodes results in a more complex signal.

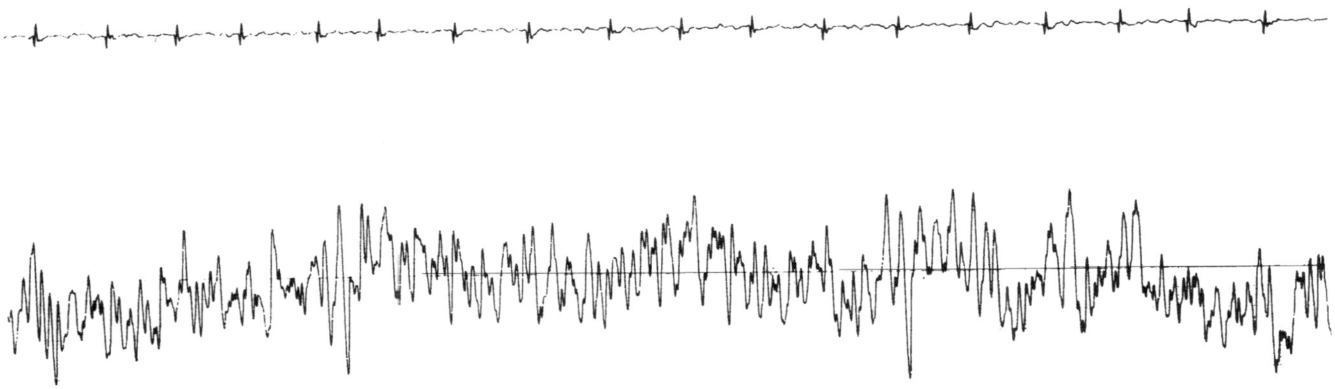

10. Intensive care instrumentation

A schematic representation of the function of an intensive care unit was given in Chapter 1. Patients under intensive care are at a critical phase of their lives and require virtually constant care from nursing staff. The constant vigilance necessary can best be provided by electronic equipment, which functions 24 hours per day, leaving nurses to devote most of their valuable time to nursing.

Since the separate electronic instruments have already been described in the previous chapters, this chapter will be very short, only describing the modifications made to instruments when used in intensive care conditions.

In general the electronic instruments which make up the intensive care system respond to such parameters as ECG, heart rate, blood pressure, body temperature and respiration. The choice of parameters to be monitored depends on the patient being observed. Often, therefore, part of the intensive care instrumentation, the bedside unit, is modular in design, providing some flexibility in the choice of parameters. By the addition or substitution of modules, the bedside unit can be adapted easily for each individual case. The choice also depends on the personal experience and ideas of special measuring systems which the medical staff may have.

Instrumentation can be specially adapted to the treatment of heart disease, as in a coronary care unit. Of course the complete unit consists not only of the necessary monitoring equipment, but also the appropriately trained personnel and emergency equipment to facilitate immediate treatment. The additional equipment of coronary care units will be described in the next chapter. In this chapter, the general approach to intensive care will be dealt with.

As already mentioned, some modular equipment is situated at the patient's bedside. These modules usually have their own display facilities and are supplied with an alarm unit. The alarm unit is often visual but positioned so that the patient himself cannot see it. An alarm is activated if certain limits are exceeded, for instance the heart rate (see next chapter).

To survey more than one patient at once, the output signals of all bedside units are carried through cables to a central desk unit or central station, so that the parameters and alarm signals of all patients are available at one central point of the intensive care unit. There are widely varying approaches to the presentation of these signals in a surveyable arrangement of oscilloscope screens, meters and graphic recorders.

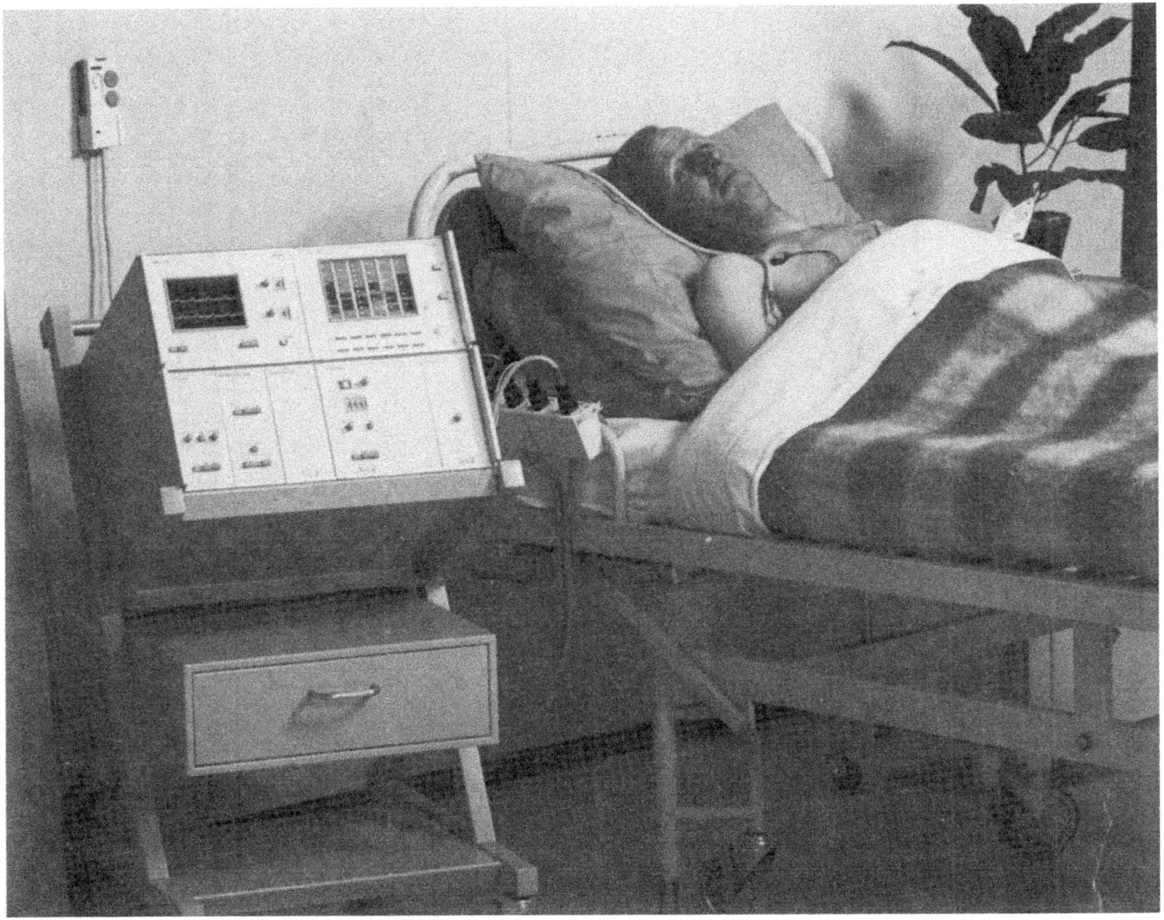

Fig. 10.1. An example of the installation of monitor bedside units.

More often, the central unit is provided with one or two multi-channel oscilloscopes for displaying the most relevant signals. One recent innovation is the use of a colour TV screen on which the signals of each patient are displayed in different colours. Depending on the location of the central desk with respect to the beds, a closed-circuit television link is also sometimes included in the intensive care unit.

In general it is not necessary to record all signals continuously, but it is imperative that every critical moment should be observed and analysed directly. For this reason some automation is incorporated in the central unit. For instance, it is possible that one ECG recorder is used to record an ECG of each patient in turn. If, however, an alarm signal is received from a certain patient, this patient needs extra attention at that moment, and the ECG recorder is switched over automatically to record from that bed. The choice of whether one or more ECGs are used depends on the expected frequency of alarms and, of course, on the number of patients connected. If more recorders are in use then the central station has the extra duty of automatically choosing the appropriate recorder.

In the event of an alarm the doctor will also be interested in the patient's ECG as it appeared immediately before the cardiac malfunction that turned on the alarm signal. This function can generally be provided by a continuous recording of the ECG on a magnetic tape loop. The length of the tape loop is such that it enables a recording of, for instance, one minute to be made. As multichannel magnetic tape recorders are used, this can be carried out simultaneously on all patients. Thus, at any given time the magnetic tape will contain the previous one minute of the patient's ECG. In the event of an alarm the tape recorder automatically writes out the ECG signal recorded in the minute leading up to that event. Instead of magnetic tape units, solid-state memories are now more commonly used. The reliability of these magnetic memories is generally much higher than magnetic tape units, as they have no moving parts.

Although the complete intensive care system may become quite complex in structure, the operation of the system is relatively simple. Still, some general remarks about actual operation should be made in order to help medical staff maintain the reliability of the unit.

To help choose which signals have to be observed continuously, the nurses must be thoroughly informed about each patient. They have to know which signal is most important or which combination of signals are most critical in determining the patient's condition. Therefore the setting of the alarm limits (see next chapter) must also be adapted to each particular case. The nurses must be fully conversant with the significance of each parameter and be familiar with the transducers in use. Also real and false alarms must be distinguished quickly, which also implies that the staff are fully acquainted with the system. Of course it is necessary to periodically test and calibrate all relevant functions of the complete instrumentation.

After an alarm has been received, necessary treatment has to be carried out immediately. This often means that within a short time additional equipment has to be installed around the patient's bed. An intensive care unit has therefore to be built in very spacious surroundings.

Since more than one piece of electronic equipment is connected to the patient in intensive care, the risk of faulty connection is increased. In other words, in order to guarantee maximum safety for the patient, a thorough knowledge of the possible dangers when working with electrical instruments is necessary for intensive care personnel. A thorough study of the last chapter of this book is therefore strongly recommended.

11. Coronary care instrumentation

As mentioned in the previous chapter, the instrumentation of a coronary care unit is specially adapted for use in the treatment of diseases of the heart, such as myocardial infarction or 'heart attack'. This means that the choice of the modules for the bedside unit is already determined by the installation of the whole system.

Some additional remarks should be made about the monitors, especially regarding their performance in a coronary care unit. The internal filters determine whether the monitor can be used only as an indicator or also as a measuring device for diagnosis.

If only monitoring facilities are necessary, the bandwidth is usually limited to 0.5 Hz–30 Hz, and often only a limited number of leads can be chosen by means of the lead selector switch. For a diagnosis the bandwidth has to be extended to 0.05 Hz–100 Hz. This can be achieved by one control designated 'monitor/diagnosis' or sometimes the low cut-off frequency is set by a control 'monitor (0.5 Hz) – diagnosis (0.05 Hz)' and the high cut-off frequency by another control 'normal (100 Hz) – damped (30 Hz)' or, in the unit illustrated, by a push-button labelled 'filter'.

The choice of these possibilities has to be made during the installation of an intensive care unit, but the choice for a coronary care unit will of course be the fullest range of possibilities adapted as much as possible to the normal cardiological requirements.

Fig. 11.1. An example of heart-rate monitor and detector.

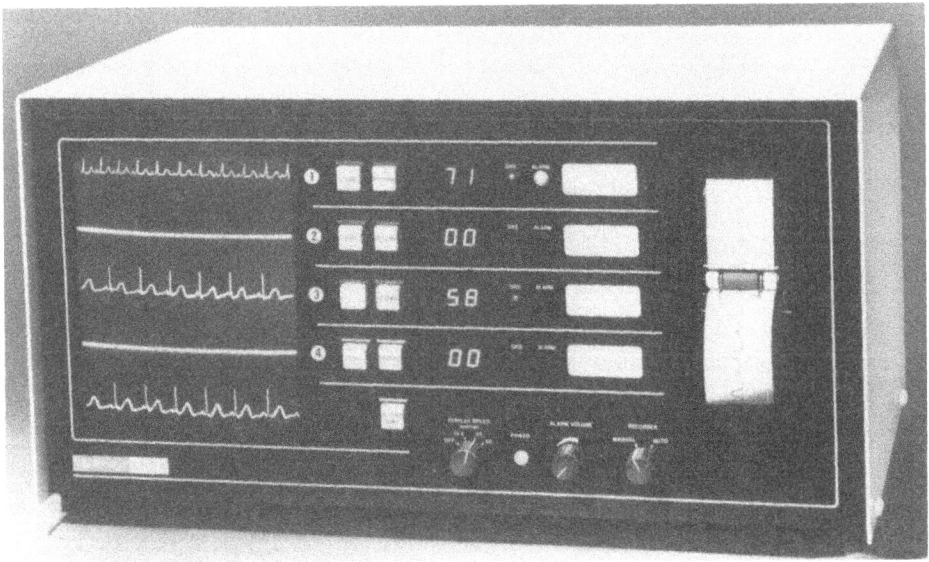

Although the heart rate can always be calculated from the ECG recording if the time scale is known, it is much easier if the average heart rate can be read directly. This can be obtained electronically by a counter circuit and displayed on a separate analogue or digital meter, or directly on the screen of the monitor. With some monitors this is achieved by means of a second trace which forms a brilliant horizontal beam whose length is related to the heart rate; on other monitors the heart rate can be displayed in digital form on the screen. The personal views of the medical and nursing staff often decide which system is preferred.

The heart-rate section, with corresponding alarm settings, of the bedside unit needs some further explanation. It is quite easy to count voltage pulses by means of an electronic circuit. Such a circuit is called a 'tachometer circuit', and the whole section is therefore called a 'cardiotachometer'. In fact, the R-waves of an ECG complex are converted into voltage pulses, with a certain amplitude and width; the original form of the R-wave is not of interest. The tachometer circuit is calibrated so that the output voltage is proportional to the number of heart beats per minute. The applied display can therefore be directly indicated in beats per minute. As the output is a voltage, this makes it possible to compare the tachometer output voltage with other adjustable voltages, which are used as upper and lower limits. A comparator circuit will give a visible or audible alarm if the tachometer output signal exceeds the preset limits. To prevent the limits being accidentally exceeded the baseline of the original ECG has to be flat. The ECG monitor is therefore often used in the 'monitor' mode.

To prevent false alarms due to artifacts such as electrode movements, the alarm is often only switched on if the heart-rate signal exceeds the preset limits during a certain period of time.

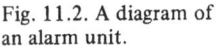

Fig. 11.2. A diagram of an alarm unit.

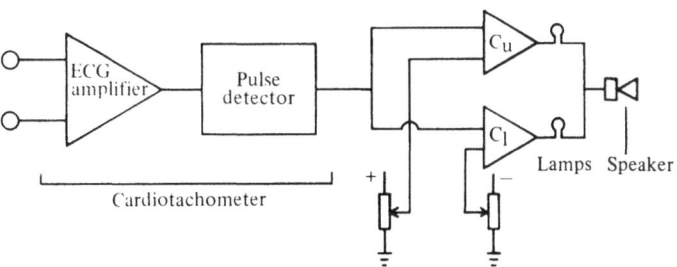

Comparators for upper and lower limits

This is effected by an internal delay circuit built into the tachometer. If false alarms still occur frequently it is very tempting to adjust the limits to lower and higher values. However, this makes the equipment worthless and it is better to spend some time searching for the cause of the artifacts.

Instead of using an ECG as an input for the cardiotachometer, the peripheral pulse wave can also be used as the input signal. In this case a plethysmographic photoelectric transducer may be used. One advantage is that now no electric contact is made with the patient, and another is that no disturbance of the tachogram will occur due to the use of a defibrillator (see further in this chapter). If the ECG amplifier is not protected against defibrillator pulses, the use of a peripheral pulse sensor is then the only way to measure the cardiac activity.

If the patient's heart is activated by an artificial pacemaker (see further in this chapter) then a peripheral pulse sensor must often be used for heart-rate detection, because some ECG amplifiers will also measure the pulses of the pacemaker. In this case the heart-rate monitor would 'take care of' the pacemaker instead of the patient. This is not the purpose of patient care. However, the newer designs of ECG monitors have suppressor circuits for pacemaker signals as well as protecting circuits for defibrillator pulses. The choice of whether an ECG or a peripheral pulse will be used as the input of the heart-rate section of the equipment then depends on the personal preference of the user.

Besides the measurements of ECG, peripheral blood flow and heart rate, which are often carried out in normal intensive care units, coronary care units usually have a measuring system for blood pressure and temperature. The transducers which can be used for measuring these physical parameters are described in detail in Chapter 5. The choice of a method for measuring the blood pressure again depends on the personal view of the user. Systems for automatic cuff inflation and microphone detection of Korotkoff sounds for blood-pressure measurement have not proved to be satisfactory in practice. Besides, this is a sampling technique and thus not suitable for continuous recording. If intra-arterial catheters with external or internal transducers are used, stringent conditions must be observed for the patient's safety. These conditions do not only apply to the blood-pressure measurement equipment itself, but also to all the measuring equipment in use in a coronary care unit. Much more attention has to be paid to all interconnections of apparatus and also to occasional use of additional equipment.

As with all oscilloscopes, the electron beam of an ECG monitor traces a path from left to right; however, in order to make comparison with paper recordings easier, ECG monitors can be made to have a right-to-left writing direction. The choice of writing direction depends on the personal taste of the user.

To complete this chapter concerning coronary care instrumentation, two more subjects will be dealt with — namely the pacemaker and the defibrillator, both pieces of electronic apparatus very commonly in use at the present time.

The pacemaker

It is possible to apply artificial stimulation to the tissue of the heart to replace its natural stimulation if this is failing to activate the heart muscle at the correct frequency. A pulsed electrical current, applied to a sensitive area of the heart, can supply artificial stimulation. It is necessary to have an adequate pulse generator available, together with leads and stimulation electrodes. The pacemaker is a specially developed design of such a stimulator.

One can distinguish between temporary and implantable pacemakers. Temporary pacemakers have been developed and are employed for short-term applications, usually less than one week. When long-term permanent pacing, perhaps over a period of years, is required, an implantable pacemaker is employed. The temporary pacemaker consists essentially of a battery-powered (to fulfil safety requirements) pulse generator and may operate in an asynchronous mode or in a demand mode. In the asynchronous mode, the current pulses are generated at a fixed, although manually adjustable, rate in the range of 50 to 150 pulses per minute. The amplitudes may also be manually controlled in the range of 0.1 to 20 mA, while the duration of each pulse is generally fixed at 1.8 ms.

In the demand mode, the pulses are only generated when the natural heart-rate falls below the preset rate of the pacemaker. In this case the pacemaker also contains an ECG amplifier which senses the ECG by means of the same electrodes as those used for stimulation. The internal pulse-generating circuit is programmed in such a way that the circuit remains inactive if an R-wave is detected within 1000 ms (1 s) of the previous R-wave, but it emits a current pulse if a longer delay than this occurs.

The stimulating electrodes are usually of the tip and ring type,

Fig. 11.3. An example of a temporary pace-maker. Note the indications for the various controllable functions: pulse amplitude (0.1 – 16 mA), rate (30–150 pulses per minute) and sensitivity for R-wave detection. A monitoring meter indicates the sensed R-wave and the pacer output. The catheter tip is connected to the — and the ring to the + output (see Fig. 11.4). When in use, the pacemaker is covered with a transparent cover to prevent accidental changing of dials.

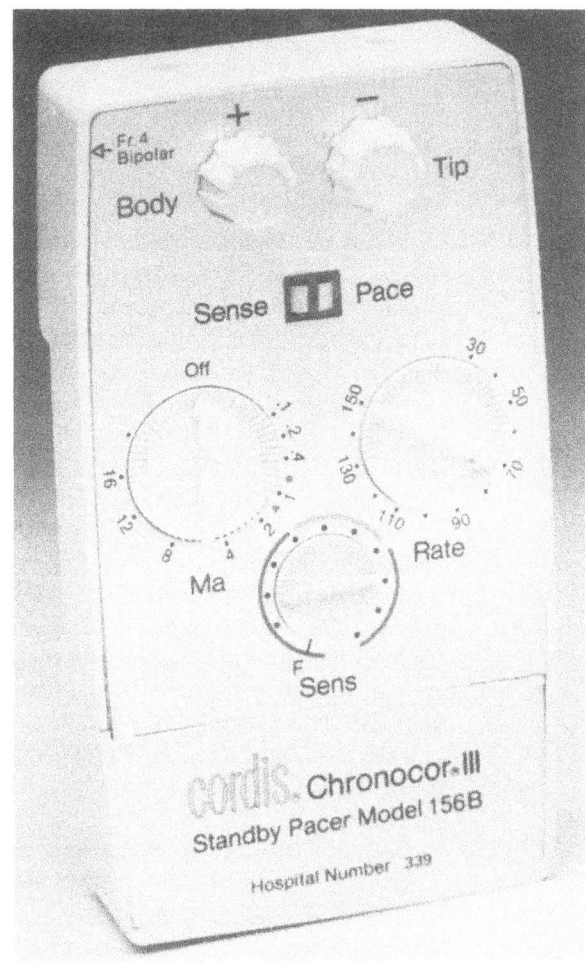

Fig. 11.4. Various types of catheter tip and ring electrodes.

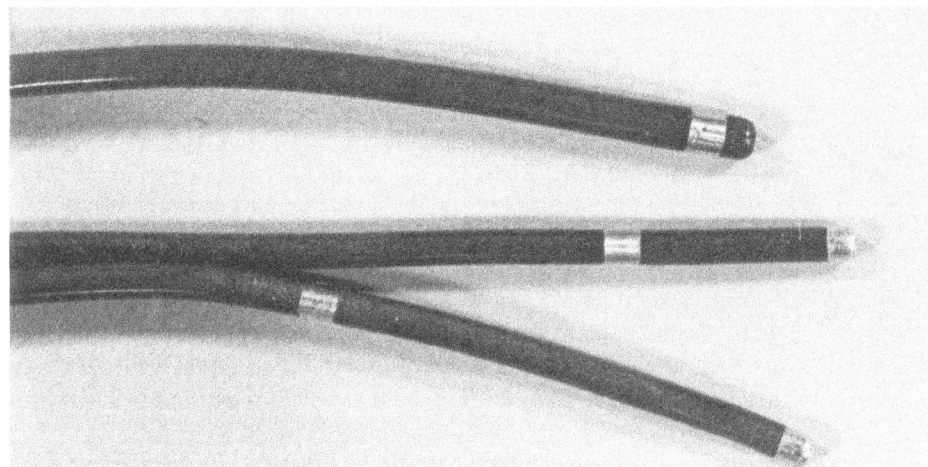

which means that the electrode lead has a platinum tip at the distal end and a platinum ring a short distance back from the tip.

A transvenous endocardial electrode is popular for temporary pacing. In this case the tip, as described above, is situated inside the ventricle of the heart. A direct contact is then made between the myocardium and the outside world; this contact demands that coronary care staff give maximum attention to ensure the patient's safety.

Care should be exercised to avoid touching the bare ends of the wires or connector at the proximal end of the leads to prevent any risk of a flow of leakage current direct to the heart (see next chapter). A few microamps may be sufficient to produce ventricular fibrillation. Furthermore, accidental movement of the electrodes should be prevented. The pacemaker must be pinned or taped directly to the patient's arm or another fixed position.

The implantable pacemakers have to fulfil the same function as the temporary types but, because they have to be employed for long periods, they are specially developed for this case. The implantable pacemaker is in fact a type of miniaturised pulse generator encased in a material which is compatible with the body tissue. The most commonly used materials are silicone rubber, epoxy resins and the metal titanium. A titanium body prevents interference with generators outside the body (diathermy units, ignition systems or microwave ovens), is impermeable to moisture, and may also act as one of the electrodes. The actual electrode lead may consist of only one insulated wire with a platinum tip.

Implantable pacemakers in common use may be divided into fixed rate and on-demand types, although other types have also been developed for special cases. In recent years, special attention has been paid to the energy supply of the pacemaker circuit. Microelectronic technology means that the electronic circuit itself may be as small as a new halfpenny or a dime, but the batteries necessary for the supply are still rather bulky. Therefore much effort is being made to find alternative long-life energy supplies.

There is also a trend to develop the circuits inside the pacemaker in such a way that it is possible to test the condition of the circuit, the batteries and the electrode impedances by measurements made outside the body.

As already mentioned in this chapter, care has to be taken with the choice of the method of measuring the heart activity of a pacemaker patient. If the heart-rate monitor also senses the pacemaker pulses, the heart rate indicated should be interpreted accordingly. In this case a plethysmographic pulse sensor has to be used or else an ECG amplifier which includes a circuit to suppress pacemaker pulses.

The defibrillator

Ventricular fibrillation is one of the most serious cardiac arrhythmias. In this case, the muscle fibres contract at random instead of in a coordinated sequence. Consequently, blood flow no longer occurs, an emergency of the first order which should be terminated within a few minutes to prevent irreversible damage to the cell metabolism of the patient, especially to the brain cells. The required synchronisation of all the fibres simultaneously can be provided by one current pulse provided by a defibrillator.

As already mentioned in Chapter 4, the defibrillator consists basically of a large capacitor, which can be charged by a power supply and discharged on command via the patient. The necessary discharge current pulse of about 5 ms duration can only be provided by a potential in the order of several thousand volts across the capacitor. The output is, as already described in Chapter 4, expressed in energy ($V \times I \times t$), thus in watt seconds or joules. Besides the control for charging the capacitor from the internal

Fig. 11.5. An implantable pacemaker with catheter electrode attached to it. Note the relatively large volume necessary for the batteries.

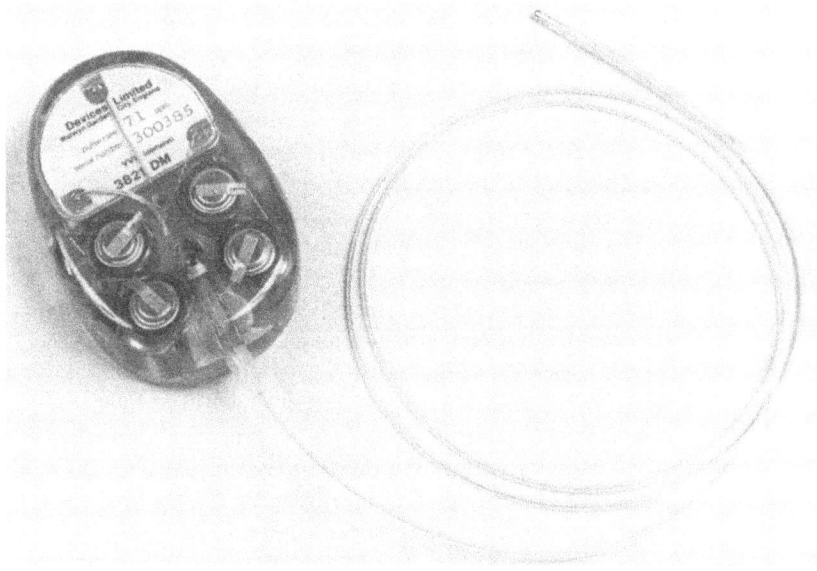

power supply, a meter is usually found on the front panel of the defibrillator labelled energy (W s or J).

Most defibrillators can store up to 400 W s, but initial attempts to defibrillate a heart are often done by lower settings of the energy adjustment. If the first current pulse is unsuccessful, the energy level is increased and a further attempt is made. It is the task of the operator to ensure that this energy is transferred to the patient. Here again, an electrode problem may occur because the electronic equipment and the patient are connected by means of electrodes (called paddles because of their shape). The electrode–patient connection is affected by an electrode impedance, which stores part of the injected energy, resulting in heat at the place of contact. In this case it is again true that the lower the electrode impedance the better, so the paddle surfaces have to be thoroughly coated with a conducting jelly and must be held firmly against the patient. Insufficient jelly or contact pressure will increase the energy losses at the place of contact, reducing the energy which is actually delivered to the patient. The same energy loss occurs if jelly is allowed to spread out over the skin between the two paddles.

The capacitor must never be discharged accidentally, neither through the patient nor through the operator, who could have the

Fig. 11.6. A diagram of defibrillator circuit and points of application of the external paddles of the defibrillator.

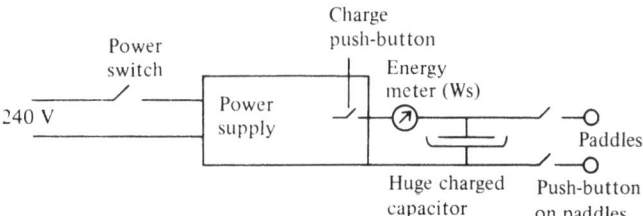

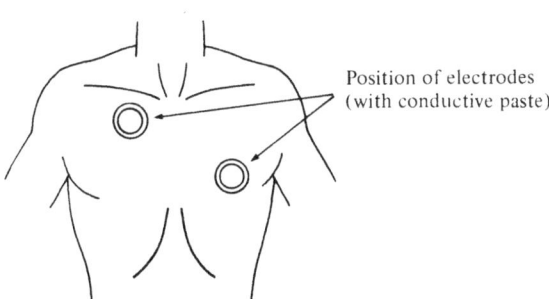

bare paddles in his hand at that moment. Safety is maximised by ensuring that the discharge is only possible when two switches, connected in series, are activated simultaneously. These push-button switches are located in the paddles in such a way that they can only be pushed when they are pressed against the patient. All other systems, for instance a foot-switch, are unsafe.

Another safety rule is that nobody should touch the patient during defibrillation. The operator should warn everyone in the vicinity to stand back at the critical moment.

During surgical exposure of the heart, interior paddles are used which can be brought directly in contact with the myocardium. Of course, the required energy level is considerably smaller than in the case of external defibrillation with so-called 'anterior—anterior' paddles.

One additional option on the defibrillator is a built-in ECG amplifier. This makes the instrument useful for treating arrhythmias other than ventricular fibrillation, such as atrial fibrillation and atrial flutter. In this case the actual current pulse cannot be delivered to the heart at any time, but only during the period of the patient's R-wave. To provide the defibrillator with this information, the presence of the R-wave has to be detected. The defibrillator does not discharge immediately when the paddle buttons are pressed, but waits after the command until the patient's next R-wave and then discharges automatically. The instrument now operates in the so-called 'synchronous mode'; without these synchronising facilities the defibrillator can only be used in the 'instantaneous mode'.

As the defibrillator is an instrument which has to operate faultlessly in the case of emergency, extreme care must be taken when using and handling it. Periodic inspections and frequent tests are absolutely necessary. It is a good practice to have a spare set of paddles conveniently available, or even a complete set of equipment in reserve. It is also worthwhile to organise regular and frequent training in sudden operation and trouble-shooting.

Fig. 11.7. A diagram of a triggered defibrillator for synchronising the defibrillator pulse with respect to the R-wave.

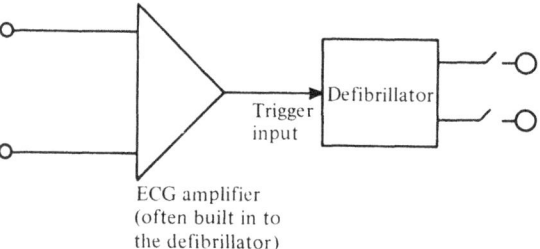

ECG amplifier
(often built in to
the defibrillator)

12. Electrical safety

As mentioned in the Preface, and also in Chapter 1, the aim of this book is to promote the safe and responsible use of electro-medical equipment, in a manner which will be of most benefit to the patient. To guide the user towards safer application and which conditions should be fulfilled to prevent possible electrical hazards, a basic knowledge of electricity is essential. The first few chapters of this book may be helpful in this respect, and re-reading of these chapters is recommended at this stage. This chapter is not only the most important one, but also the most difficult to grasp.

Some recommendations to ensure the safe application of various items of equipment have been given in the corresponding chapters. Nevertheless it is useful to bring all these safety require-ments together in this final chapter, where they may be examined from a more general point of view.

Broadly speaking, there are two sources of electrical hazard encountered in a medical environment, those arising from static electricity and those arising from the use of mains power supplies.

Static electricity
Static electricity is not, in fact, used in electromedical instrumen-tation. It still, however, presents a threat to patient safety. As already mentioned in Chapter 2, nylon clothing may generate high voltages which can give rise to sparks, especially in dry atmospheres. It is easy to imagine the hazard that this presents, particularly in the presence of certain explosive gases, such as ether or cyclopropane, sometimes used in anaesthesia.

A hazard of a secondary nature may also arise from the presence of static electricity. Should a patient or member of staff experience a static discharge in the form of a spark, their sudden reaction may result in many types of accident. Bottles may be knocked over, perhaps spilling their contents over equipment, or patient-connecting leads may be accidentally disconnected.

These hazards arising from static electricity are always present where materials which aid the build-up of static charges are used. It is now standard practice for operating theatre staff to wear cotton clothing, in preference to the newer synthetic materials. Operating theatres are built with conducting floors, and trolleys are fitted with conducting rubber tyres. Fortunately, explosive gases are now no longer widely used in anaesthesia and the hazard is now less than in the past.

Mains-associated hazards

Even when the hazards arising from static electricity are successfully eliminated, hazards arising from the use of equipment which requires an electrical mains supply still remain. The rest of this chapter will be devoted to this topic.

In general, it is the flow of electrical current through a patient which presents the hazard. As already described in Chapter 4, the value of current in a circuit depends on the voltage of the electrical supply, 240 V, 100 V or 220 V a.c. r.m.s. (see p. 16), in the case of a mains supply, and also on the total impedance of the circuit. This may consist of the impedance of the patient and perhaps two connecting electrodes. It is thus difficult to give general values of voltage which may be fatal, and it is found that current flow through the patient is the only useful parameter, as indicated in Table 12.1. These current values are expressed on a scale ranging from the threshold of sensation, through muscle stimulation to tissue damage, and were determined by connecting a 50 Hz voltage to the chest of a dog for 1 second. Unfortunately, the heart is particularly sensitive to current at this frequency, and from this point of view the choice of 50 Hz for the mains supply is a bad one.

When experiments are carried out to determine the current sensitivity of the heart, it can be seen that even currents in the microamp range passing through the most sensitive part of the heart may cause fibrillation and hence are dangerous. In this chapter examples will be given of patient-instrumentation systems where such small currents may easily flow through the heart, often arising from unexpected leakage currents flowing through connections between the equipment and the patient. Safety regulations must therefore be drawn up to prevent excessive leakage currents.

An internationally accepted maximum limit is 10 μA for each patient-lead or connection.

Table 12.1. *Effect of current flow*

Current	Effect
1 mA	Threshold of sensation.
16 mA	Muscle contraction, cannot let go of supply.
50 mA	Pain, possible loss of consciousness, mechanical damage, heart and respiration still function.
100 mA—3 A	Ventricular fibrillation, respiratory paralysis, severe burns.

Fuses. Before more specific cases of safe use of electromedical equipment are discussed, a general point of misunderstanding must be clarified. It concerns the use of fuses in electronic equipment and in power lines. These fuses have no direct function in preventing current flow through the patient. The reason that these fuses are connected in series with the circuits is to prevent the overheating that may arise if short circuits occur. The fuse breaks the circuit if a certain high current flow is exceeded and so prevents damage to the circuit itself. However, before a fuse 'blows', a large current has already flowed. This means that a fuse provides only relatively slow protection against high currents, sufficient protection for most electronic circuits but not enough for patients. More stringent current-limiting techniques have to be used in these circumstances.

The voltage which is available at the wall-outlet socket is an alternating voltage, as already described in Chapter 2. This means that one of the poles of the outlet, the so-called 'live' or 'power line', is periodically positive and negative with respect to the other pole, the so-called 'neutral line'. This neutral line is connected to a large electrode which is driven into the ground at the power station or transformer house. This then means that at these places the voltage of the neutral line is exactly zero with respect to the earth potential.

The wall-outlet is connected to the power station by means of cables, or power lines, through which the current flows. Current may be drawn from the outlet, and also from others which are connected to the power station by means of the same cable. Although power lines or cables are made from highly conducting materials, usually copper, they still have a finite resistance. This means that a voltage difference is created between both ends of the power line, the value of the voltage depending on the resistance of the line and the total current flowing through it. As a consequence, the voltage of the neutral line is not zero with respect to the local earth, but may reach values of up to 10 V a.c. r.m.s. Thus both the power line and the neutral line carry an alternating voltage with respect to the local earth, which can be contacted through the water supply or perhaps through a damp floor.

It will now be obvious that using equipment with a metal case and a two-prong plug may be very dangerous. If one of the leads of the power line accidentally makes contact with this metal case someone could easily make contact with this lead and, whether it is 'live' or 'neutral', be subjected to a dangerous source of current.

The advice which is often given to turn a two-prong plug round in the two-slot outlet if one 'feels' a voltage when touching the case of an apparatus is thus dangerous nonsense. It is obvious that two-slot outlets and apparatus with two-prong plugs should never be used in a hospital. In some countries two-prong plugs have been forbidden, even for household use. In others it is impossible to plug in the wrong way as the prongs are 'staggered'. This practice should be adopted internationally.

The problem of accidental contact between a power line and the metal case of a piece of equipment giving rise to a dangerous condition has long been solved. The solution is quite simple, namely to connect the metal case of the apparatus to the local earth. Then in principle a voltage can never be created between the metal case and the local earth of the water supply, central heating, or whatever is used.

Earthing of metal cases is simple, because a local earth line is provided in earthed sockets and contacts the plug by means of a third slot. Of course three-prong (earthed) plugs have to be used for connecting electrical equipment using a three-lead power cord, one live, one neutral and one earth lead. Sometimes additional earth leads are also used to connect equipment more securely to the local earth.

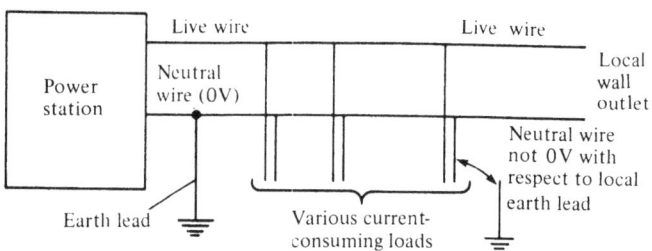

Fig. 12.1. A diagram of mains wiring with local and remote earth lead.

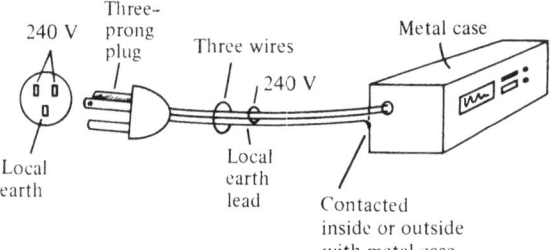

Fig. 12.2. A schematic representation of three-prong plug with corresponding three-lead power cord for earthing the applied equipment.

Note that now a new danger may occur; the operator of an instrument now relies on the fact that the device is earthed, but this is not the case if the earth lead has broken within the three-wire power cord. These power cords must therefore be tested regularly and if any fault is observed in a plug or the power cord itself, a replacement must be provided. It will also be obvious that an adaptor must never be disconnected by pulling on the power cord; this can cause damage to the wires. One cannot be too careful!

IEC Regulations. All electrical equipment which is intended for use in medical environments should comply with certain safety requirements, usually determined by the government of the country in which it is to be used. For their guidance, the International Electrotechnical Commission, abbreviated to IEC, has made certain safety rules which every piece of electrical equipment should satisfy. In general, these rules concern the construction, admissible leakage currents and insulation requirements.

Particular rules have been drafted for electromedical equipment, drawn up by an IEC sub-commission called IEC 62A, installed in 1968. One of the big problems for this commission has been dealing with non-medical electrical equipment which is used in hospitals. Things like vacuum cleaners and lighting circuits, which are not designed for use in hospitals, often cause potentially dangerous situations. The IEC 62A is at present making rules which are also applicable to this more common type of electrical equipment. It is therefore advisable to apply these rules now if new installations are built, even before they are internationally

Fig. 12.3. A broken earth lead results in an extremely dangerous situation with respect to leakage currents due to touching an apparatus.

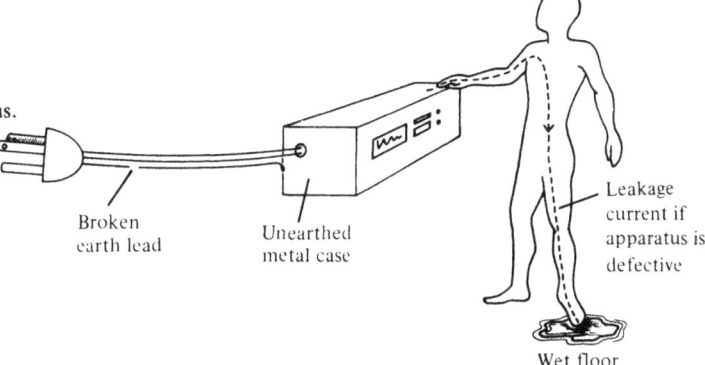

Broken earth lead

Unearthed metal case

Leakage current if apparatus is defective

Wet floor

accepted. This is of the greatest importance for the patient's safety, and thus for the patient's life.

The IEC has attempted to classify equipment into various types. Class I consists of mains-powered equipment contained within a metal case. Instruments may also be found with insulated cases where it is impossible to make contact with a live part, since the wires inside the device have an insulating coating of their own. This kind of equipment, called double-insulated, can be identified by the sign □ . An electric shaver, for instance, belongs to this class, which is the only class which may be used with a two-wire power cord. These pieces of equipment fall within Class II, in terms of IEC standards.

A third class of electrical equipment, IEC Class III, includes equipment which does not need a power cord at all because it is battery-powered. These are the safest kinds of device because no leakage currents to earth can occur and the supply voltages are in general much smaller than the mains supply.

Returning to Class I equipment, apparatus with earthed metal cases and in principle safe for application in the biomedical field, can still be dangerous if this equipment is used in combination with other equipment. This other equipment need not necessarily be intended for biomedical use, it could be a bed light for instance. The next example shows a common situation, the danger of which is not always appreciated.

A patient is connected to an earthed instrument by means of electrodes or a saline-filled catheter. Usually the patient is also

Fig. 12.4. Schematic diagram of Class II, double-insulated apparatus.

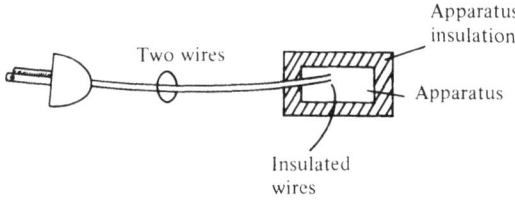

Fig. 12.5. Battery-operated equipment can not provide leakage currents to earth.

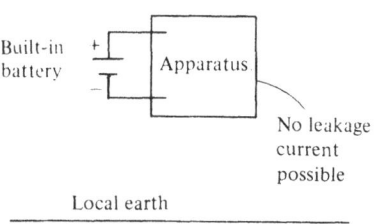

earthed by means of one of these connections. If a bed light mounted above the patient has poor internal insulation because of the intense heat of the bulb damaging the internal insulation, it may happen that metal parts of the bed light have a voltage with respect to earth. This means that a current will flow to earth through the patient as soon as he touches this light. The same thing can happen if a nurse touches the patient and the badly-insulated light at the same time. The currents which flow under these circumstances are often greater than the limiting value of 10 μA, and in many cases may result in the sudden onset of fibrillation.

A less obvious hazard is presented by any piece of mains-powered equipment, whether this has a faulty insulation or not. As mentioned in Chapter 5, any capacitance presents a conducting path for alternating current, and these currents pass between the closely-bound conductors within a mains lead. Normally these leakage currents are returned safely to earth via the earth connection in the mains plug. Should this become disconnected, however, and the patient make contact with the case of such a device, the mains leakage currents will pass to earth through the body of the patient. Thus it is not necessary for an insulation fault to occur to render the equipment potentially dangerous. This can occur by a faulty earth connection alone.

The use of specially designed mains isolation transformers, which provide a floating mains supply, is often believed to remove the danger from leakage currents. However some leakage current

Fig. 12.6. Typical example of leakage current as a result of bad insulation inside a bed light.

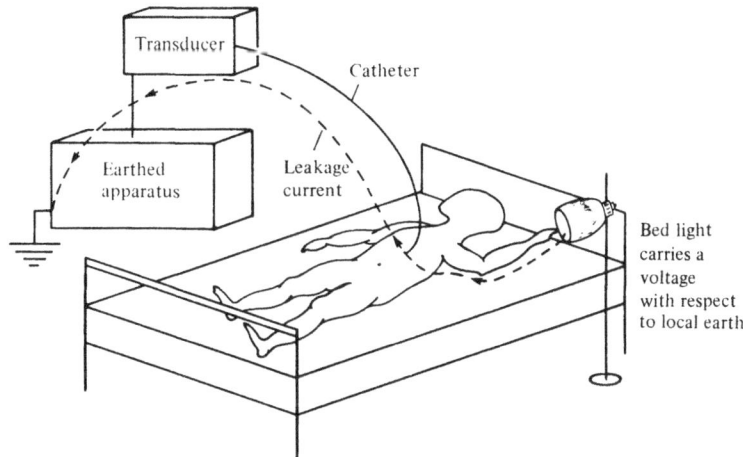

will still flow to earth by way of the transformer capacitance.

Another problem which may occur with Class I instruments arises when two pieces of equipment are used simultaneously, both having their own connection between the patient and earth. If each instrument is supplied by a three-prong plug in a different wall outlet, one on the left and one on the right side of the bed for instance, then a current may flow through the patient by way of the two earth leads if the earths of the two wall outlets are not exactly equal in potential. Although a local ground connection must always be 0 V, thus making it in principle impossible that a voltage can be present between two earth connections, it can still happen that an earth lead may carry a certain potential. The reason for this is that a piece of equipment may have some degree of internal short circuit without blowing a fuse, which means that a leakage current flows through the earth lead. As the internal resistance of the earth lead will never be exactly zero, especially if the earth lead is relatively long, the leakage current will create a voltage across the lead.

In older hospitals especially, where various structural alterations have taken place with consequent changes in the electrical wiring, the different interconnections of earth leads are often not clearly

Fig. 12.7. The use of two separate wall outlets can result in a leakage current between the different earth leads.

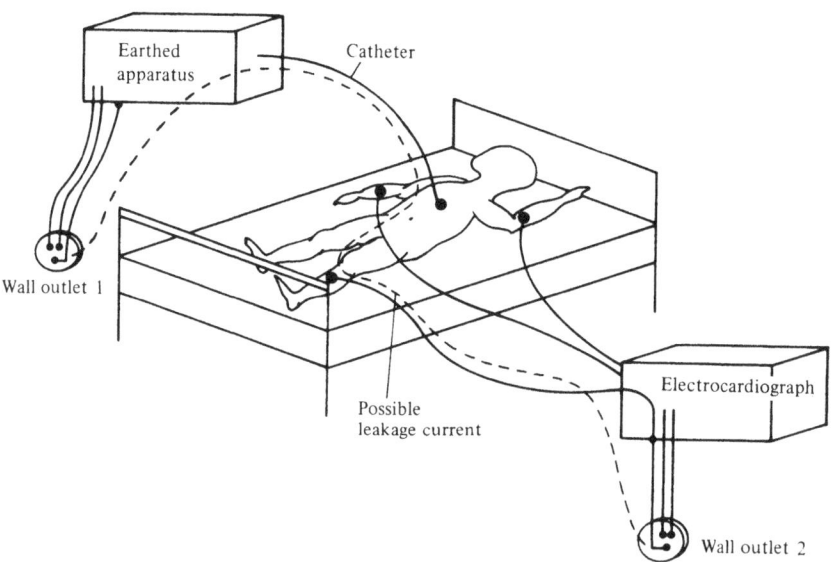

Earthed apparatus

Catheter

Wall outlet 1

Electrocardiograph

Possible leakage current

Wall outlet 2

indicated. This means that the earth connection of one wall outlet may accidentally carry a voltage due to the use of another piece of equipment, for instance a vacuum cleaner, somewhere else in that room or even an adjacent room. In this way, the earth of one wall outlet may easily have a certain voltage with respect to the earth of another wall outlet, resulting in a leakage current from one earth to the other. Leakage currents exceeding the limiting value of 10 μA are very commonly the result of this effect, which may result in a ventricular fibrillation. The only remedy is never to use two separately spaced wall outlets. At each bed a complete set of at least four wall outlets with one common earth plate should be available, and only this set of wall outlets used for all the electrical equipment in use on the patient in that bed.

Furthermore, all metal objects in the neighbourhood of the bed should be earthed by means of a connection to the same earth plate, which can be seen as a central earth for that particular bed. This earth is usually called a 'star-point'. Each bed with its surrounding equipment needs its own star-point. Additional equipment occasionally used near a patient should never be plugged into a wall outlet which is not part of the star-point circuit for that bed. This means that at least one spare wall outlet has to be available at each bedside. This also prevents the necessity for using extension cables, also to be condemned from the point of view that they may impede nurses, causing them to trip or stumble. Extension cables are also not allowed in medical

Fig. 12.8. Recommended installation of equipment around a bed with only one star-point.

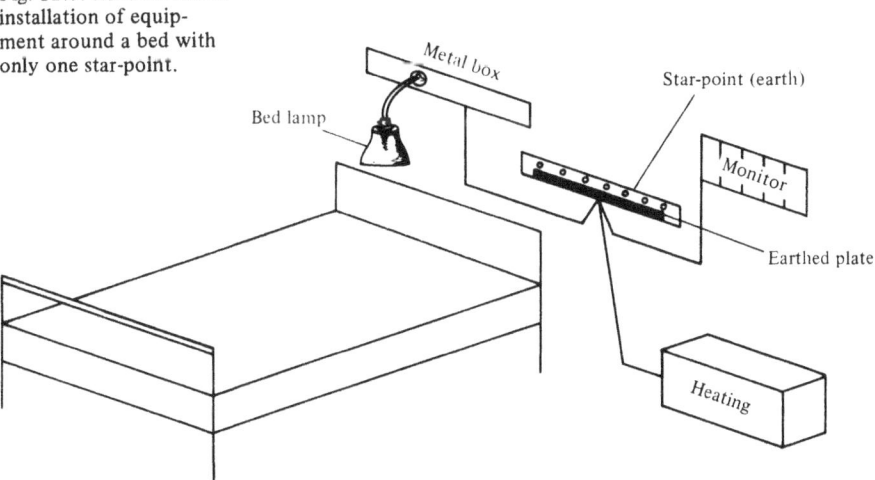

care rooms, since their use usually implies a plug connection on the floor. Because plug connections are usually not watertight, this creates a dangerous situation if liquids are accidentally spilled.

The best approach to the prevention of leakage current through the patient is the use of instruments in which each patient lead is unable to draw currents larger than 1 or 2 μA. This is especially so in the case of leads which make direct connection with the patient's heart, such as pacemaker leads or saline-filled catheters. With this type of equipment, the patient should not be earthed. Measuring equipment which fulfils these requirements uses isolation amplifiers in the input stages. These amplifiers can be bought as complete units and may be used to increase the safety of older equipment, or alternatively they may be built into new equipment. The principle is very simple and is based on the fact that signals can be transmitted by means other than electrically conducting wires.

An electrical voltage can be transformed, for instance, into a

Fig. 12.9. Do not use open connections, as in the case of extensions where moisture may cause a short-circuit.

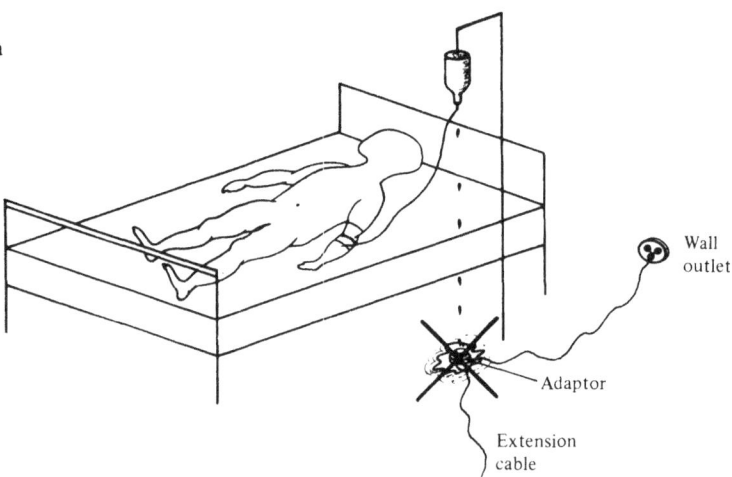

Fig. 12.10. A diagram of an isolation amplifier set-up.

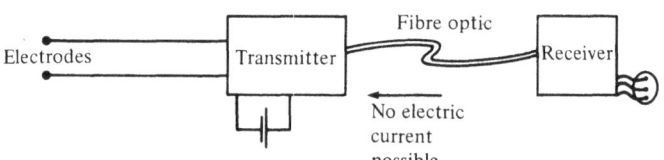

light signal in such a way that the light intensity is proportional to the amplitude of the voltage. This modulated light signal can then be transmitted through a fibre optic light guide and received by a light-sensitive device which again transforms it into an electrical signal of the same pattern as the original. This means that near-perfect insulation is achieved between transmitter and receiver, in which case the receiver may be supplied by the mains as a piece of Class I equipment. The transmitter should then be supplied by batteries.

Another approach which can be used for the transmission of signals is the use of a high-frequency carrier. This system can also be used for transmitting the necessary power for the supply of the signal transmitter, using a specially designed high-frequency transformer which has a high impedance at the frequency of the mains supply.

In both cases no leakage current can flow through the patient to earth because the isolating properties of the amplifier block all such currents.

As many instruments are not equipped with built-in isolation amplifiers, a system in which the patient is earthed has to be frequently used. If this is necessary, then extreme care must be taken when connecting more earthed equipment to the patient, as already mentioned in this chapter.

One more example illustrates that error on the part of the operator is often the reason that safety rules are disregarded. This is the case if a surgical diathermy unit is used in combination with other electromedical equipment, for instance an ECG heart-rate monitor. Usually the patient lies on a buttock plate, which is

Fig. 12.11. With a combination of an electro-cautery unit and another electromedical apparatus, only the earth lead of the electro-surgery unit may be attached to the patient.

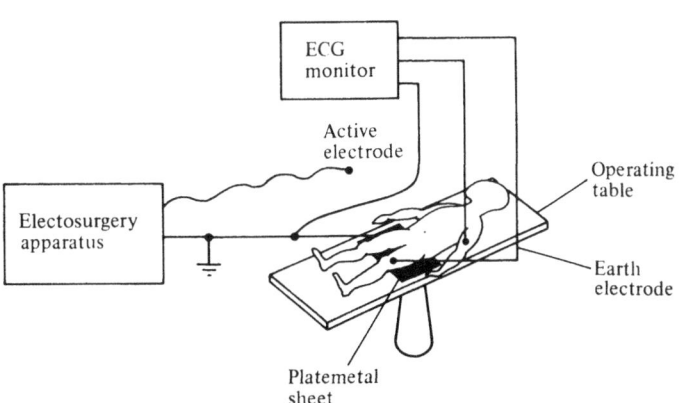

connected to the earth terminal of the corresponding unit. At the same time the patient is often earthed via the ECG ground electrode. During electrosurgery a large current flows to earth through the buttock plate. If, however, the connection between the plate and earth should break, then the large current will flow through the ECG earth lead. This will certainly result in severe burning of the patient at the place of contact of the ECG earth electrode because its surface is too small to carry the current without heating up. To prevent this, the ECG earth lead should not be connected to the patient, but should be connected to the earth terminal of the electrosurgery unit.

Modern electrosurgery apparatus is isolated from the earth, to prevent the earth problem mentioned above. Only in such apparatus may the ECG earth lead be connected to the patient.

In general, this example illustrates that electromedical equipment should not only be earthed at only one star-point, but there should also be only one earth lead between the patient and the star-point. This rule of patient single-earthing will prevent various hazards and is also useful for preventing disturbance of the measured signals by mains interference.

The hazards described in this chapter are all of the type in which the people who operate the electromedical equipment play a major role. Care in the connection of leads and power cords, and in the interconnection of equipment, can prevent many hazards. Some of the dangers are the result of the electrical installation as a whole, to which changes cannot easily be made. Taking these preset conditions into account, however, medical staff have the responsibility for allowing a certain situation or not. The following rules should be a starting point in any discussion of whether a certain situation is safe or not.

(1) Only earthed wall outlets should be present in medical care rooms of hospitals, and consequently only three-prong plugs should be used to connect electromedical equipment.

(2) Each patient must have his or her own block of wall outlets with one earthed star-point. All apparatus necessary for this patient may only be connected to these wall-outlets.

(3) All metal parts around a patient must be connected to the corresponding star-point.

(4) The patient should only be connected with one single lead to the star-point earth.

(5) Never use extension cables.

(6) Be careful with power cables. Never pull the cable, only the plug, when disconnecting the equipment.

(7) Ask for a regular test of power cables and equipment by the technical staff.

(8) If possible, use isolated amplifiers.

(9) Abandon all synthetic clothing to prevent the generation of static electricity.

(10) Always use your common-sense in all things concerned with electromedical instrumentation. If a situation looks potentially dangerous, ask for the opinion of a technically quali-fied person.

Index

accelerometer, for measuring tremor, 62

accumulators, 6; connected in series or in parallel, 8, 9; maximum voltage of, 8; miniature sealed, 6−7; recharging of, 7

accuracy, of electronic instruments, 2−3; effect on, of relation between electrode impedance and input inpedance, 87−8

action potentials, of single muscle fibres, measured with needle electrodes, 99

air, as insulator, 27

alarm units, 102, 104, 107−8; setting limits for, 105

amperes (milliamperes, microamperes), units of electric current, 22, 23

amplification factor (gain), 68, 69; temperature and, 78

amplifiers, 68−9; capacitive coupling of, with mains, 72−4; connections of, 71−2; differential, 74−6; frequency band of, 69; high-frequency signals interfering with, 77−8; isolated, 124−5, transistors in, 69−71

amplitude, of voltage waveform, 14

analogue representation of signals, 79

anode (positive pole), 6, 9−10

atrial fibrillation, atrial flutter: use of defibrillator for, 114

batteries, dry, 7−8; connected in series or in parallel, 8, 9; for implantable pacemakers, 111, 112; maximum voltage of, 8

battery-operated apparatus, safer than mains-operated, 25, 26, 120

block diagrams, 2

blood: flow of electric current in ions of (calcium, potassium, sodium), 20, 24−5, 27; measurement of pH and carbon dioxide content of, 56

blood flow: measurement of, by plethysmography, 60, and by photoplethysmography, 63, 108; measurement of velocity of, electromagnetically, 65, and by ultra-sound, 66−7

blood pressure, measured by strain gauge at outer end or tip of catheter inserted into circulation, 60−2, 108

brain, voltages generated in, *see* electroencephalogram

bridge circuit, 57

capacitance, measured in farads, 40

capacitors, storing electric charges, 39−40; acting as filters, 42−3; block direct current, conduct alternating current, 42; combinations of resistors and, for separating voltages of various frequencies, 43−4; coupling between mains and, 72−4; defibrillators as, 40−1, 112

cardiotachometer, 107; ECG as input for, 107−8; peripheral pulse wave as input for, 108

cassette recorders, for storing electrical signals, 85

catheterisation, cardiac, 60

catheters: intra-arterial, for monitoring of blood pressure and temperature, 60−2, 108; of pacemakers, 110

cathode (negative pole), 9−10

cathode-ray tubes, in oscilloscopes, 80, 81, 82

ceramics, as insulators, 27

circuit diagrams: for battery, switch, and lamp, 21; for bridge configuration, 57; for defibrillator, 41, 113; with double- and single-pole switches, 33; for earthed apparatus with mains supply, and non-earthed apparatus with battery supply, 25; for filters, 44, 45; integrated, 71; for lamps connected in series and in parallel, 22; for measurement of current, 36; for measurement of resistance, 56; for potentiometer, 38; for transistor amplifier, 70; for voltage divider, 37

circuits, electrical, 21; integrated, in amplifier, 71

coagulative apparatus: high-frequency signals from, may affect amplifiers, 77

coils of conducting wire, electromagnetic effects in, 38−9

For EU product safety concerns, contact us at Calle de José Abascal, 56–1°,
28003 Madrid, Spain or eugpsr@cambridge.org.

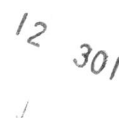